MEDICAL INTERNET OF THINGS (M-IOT) - ENABLING TECHNOLOGIES AND EMERGING APPLICATIONS

Edited by **Hamed Farhadi**

Medical Internet of Things (m-IoT) - Enabling Technologies and Emerging Applications
http://dx.doi.org/10.5772/intechopen.71858
Edited by Hamed Farhadi

Contributors

Hari Shankar Singh, Weitao Xu, Guohao Lan, Nafiseh Shariati, Dave Zachariah, Johan Karlsson, Mats Bengtsson, Julang Ying, Kaveh Pahlavan, Liyuan Xu, Thierry Edoh, Sergey Kirillov, Aleksandr Kirillov, Yuri Kaganovich, Michael Pecht, Vitalii Yakimkin, Mojtaba Fallahpour

First published in London, United Kingdom, 2019 by IntechOpen
IntechOpen is the global imprint of INTECHOPEN LIMITED, registered in England and Wales, registration number: 11086078, The Shard, 25th floor, 32 London Bridge Street
London, SE19SG – United Kingdom
Printed in Croatia

British Library Cataloguing-in-Publication Data
A catalogue record for this book is available from the British Library

Additional hard copies can be obtained from orders@intechopen.com

Medical Internet of Things (m-IoT) - Enabling Technologies and Emerging Applications , Edited by Hamed Farhadi
p. cm.
Print ISBN 978-1-78985-091-8
Online ISBN 978-1-78985-092-5

For EU product safety concerns:
IN TECH d.o.o., Prolaz Marije Krucifikse Kozulić 3, 51000 Rijeka, Croatia,
info@intechopen.com or visit our website at intechopen.com.

Meet the editor

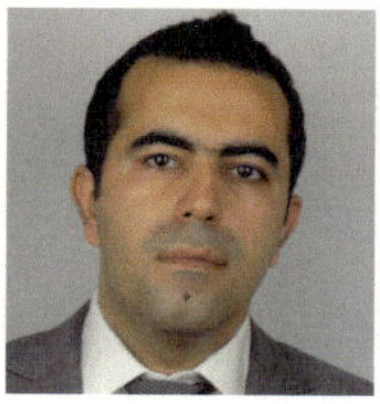

Hamed Farhadi is a Researcher at Ericsson Research, Stockholm, Sweden. He is also a Researcher at KTH Royal Institute of Technology (KTH), Stockholm, Sweden. Dr. Farhadi received his PhD degree from KTH Royal Institute of Technology, Stockholm, Sweden in 2014. He was a Postdoctoral Research Fellow at Harvard University, Cambridge, MA, USA in 2016, and a Researcher at Chalmers University of Technology, Gothenburg, Sweden in 2015. His research interests mainly lie in statistical signal processing and machine learning for a broad range of applications including wireless healthcare systems, micro-robotic surgery, clinical data analysis, and wireless information networks. He has been the recipient of several academic awards including the best paper award of IEEE International Conference on Acoustics, Speech and Signal Processing (ICASSP) in 2014. Dr. Farhadi was the co-chair of IEEE International Symposium on Medical Information and Communication Technology (ISMICT) in 2015.

Contents

Preface

The recent developments in biomedical sensors, wireless communication systems, and information networks are transforming the conventional healthcare systems. The transformed healthcare systems are enabling distributed healthcare services to patients who may not be co-located with the healthcare providers, providing early diagnoses, and reducing the cost in the healthcare section. The developments in medical internet of things (m-IoT) would enable a range of applications, including remote health monitoring through medical-grade wearables to provide homecare for elderlies; virtual doctor-patient interaction to have any time and place access to medical professionals; wireless endoscopic examination; and remotely operated robotic surgery to extend the access to highly skilled surgeons. Wireless body area networks (WBAN) are key enablers of these transformations. These networks connect sensors and actuators to external processing units, which could be placed on the surface of the patient's body or implanted inside the body to connect specific sensors and/or actuators inside, on, and around the body to the data collection points. The success of these networks highly relies on the advent of low-power, low-delay, reliable, and low-cost wireless connectivity solutions.

This book covers recent developments in wireless healthcare systems to provide an insight to the technological solutions for wireless body area networks, and emerging applications of medical internet of things and wireless healthcare systems. The book starts with a chapter on medical internet of things (m-IoT) for emergency medical care services. The chapter discusses the challenges facing the emergency medical care service delivery in the public healthcare system and presents an IoT-based emergency medical care service delivery system. The results of conducted field experiments are presented in the chapter. The book continues with the following chapters on body area networks, which are enabling technology of medical IoT systems.

Chapter 2 discusses antenna design limitations and challenges for wireless body area networking, where evaluating the antenna's performance near the human body is emphasized. The chapter presents several antenna miniaturization techniques that can be used to reduce the antennas' dimension. The chapter investigates the performance of a short-range communication system between wearable antennas and a remote node using IEEE 802.11g wireless networking protocol. The antenna design for multiple input multiple output (MIMO) systems is further discussed in Chapter 3, where the focus is on cellular communication systems. The impact of user proximity on antenna performance is investigated in this chapter.

Wireless energy transfer to devices or specific areas in/around the body is a key technology to enable a convenient source of energy for devices in body area networks and also to perform specific medical treatments. Chapter 4 addresses the topic of wireless energy transfer to specific areas inside the body. The chapter addresses the optimization of spatial power distribution generated by an array of transmitting elements for ultrasound hyperthermia cancer treatment as a motivating example. The signal design problem consists of optimizing the power distribution across the tumor and healthy tissue regions, respectively. The models that are used in the optimization problem are, however, invariably subject to errors. To combat such unknown model errors, a robust signal design framework is presented in the chapter that can take the uncertainty into account using a worst-case design approach.

With the rapid development of embedded technology and mobile computing, a growing number of wearable devices have been used by consumers. As the number of wearable devices belonging to the same user increases rapidly, secure pairing between legitimate devices becomes an important problem in body area networks. Chapter 5 presents a novel gait-based shared key generation system that assists two devices to generate a common secure key by exploiting the user's unique walking pattern, which is common among different wearable devices. The chapter supports the effectiveness of the proposed scheme by presenting the results from experimental studies.

The number of sensors mounted on smart phones and wearable devices that can measure and communicate local information from around the body area is increasing. This would enable hybrid methods to acquire situational awareness relying on heterogeneous types of information sources. Specifically, the obtained information from multiple types of sensors mounted on different devices around the body can be exploited for localization purposes. This could possibly provide more accurate, more reliable, and cost-effective navigation systems. Chapter 6 presents different sensors in wearable devices that can be used for localization purposes and investigates the accuracy of the localization techniques based on each of these sensors.

Chapter 7 is dedicated to body area networks for remote cardiac preventive monitoring. The chapter presents methods, models, and computational algorithms that are developed for a sample remote cardiac system to operate on remote clusters based on information that is received from portable ECG recorders. Computational kernels of preventive monitoring are presented in the chapter, which include several interacting automata that can be used for the prediction of heart failure. The chapter discusses how cloud computing clusters can support low-cost ultra-portable recorders to enable preventive health monitoring systems.

The book provides an overview of key enabling techniques and possible applications of body area networks. The book can be used by researchers, medical professionals, business owners, entrepreneurs, and engineers for an insight about the potential opportunities in developing solutions based on body area networks for future remote healthcare systems. The book has been the result of the effort of several authors with diverse technical backgrounds who are experts in medical science and engineering and contributed to different chapters of the book. The editor would like to use this opportunity to thank all the authors who have contributed to this book for their valuable inputs. In addition, the editor would like to thank the publication team at IntechOpen publisher who facilitated the publication process of the present book. The editor specially thanks the publication manager Ms. Romina Skomersic for all her valuable help.

Dr. Hamed Farhadi
Experienced Researcher
Ericsson Research
Stockholm, Sweden

Chapter 1

Internet of Things in Emergency Medical Care and Services

Thierry Edoh

Additional information is available at the end of the chapter

http://dx.doi.org/10.5772/intechopen.76974

Abstract

Emergency care is a critical area of medicine whose outcomes are influenced by the time, availability, and accuracy of contextual information. In addition, the success of emergency care depends on the quality and accuracy of the information received during the emergency call and data collected during the emergency transportation. The success of a follow medical treatment at an emergency care unit depends too on data collected during the two phases: emergency call and transport. However, most information received during an emergency-call is inaccurate and the process of information collection, storage, processing, and retrieval, during an emergency-transportation, is remaining manual and time-consuming. Emergency doctors mostly lack patient's health records and base the medical treatment on a set of collected information including information provided by the patient or his relatives. Hence, the emergency care delivery is more patient-centered than patient-centric information. Wireless body area network and Internet of Technology (IoT) enable accurate collection of data and are increasingly used in medical applications. This chapter discusses the challenges facing the emergency medical care services delivery, especially in the developing countries. It presents and discusses an IoT platform for a patient-centric-information-based emergency care services delivery. The study is focused on a case of road traffic injury. Results of conducted experiments are discussed.

Keywords: emergency medical care, Internet of Health Things, road congestion, pervasive/ubiquitous computing, road traffic injury

1. Introduction

Road traffic injuries are, according to the WHO report on the topic, the leading causes of death worldwide. Over 1.2 million of individuals died each year on the road [1]. "Road traffic injuries (RTI) are on increasing in developing countries. Healthcare facilities are poorly equipped to provide the needed services." [2]. Efforts are made over the past years to improve the emergency care services delivery in the developing countries. Emergency services policies and training programs for emergency providers have been implemented, though, these programs are still facing challenges in the training [3]. The developing countries are facing further challenges beyond the weak training. However, developing countries lack medical transport system. In 2002, Razzak and Kellermann carried out a study [4] and found out that the lack of medical transport is a common issue facing the most of healthcare systems in the developing world; the authors, further, state that "The provision of timely treatment during life-threatening emergencies is not a priority for many health systems in developing countries."

Previous works conducted in 2016 and 2017 in the sub-Saharan African countries have revealed that most healthcare systems have partially improved the medical transport issues by acquiring a few numbers of ambulances. However, this fact does not completely meet the issues facing the emergency transportation. The roads are in bad state and though lead to massive time-wasting, with the high risk of medical complication or death.

In [5–7], the authors have found out that electronic medical records (EMR) have the potential to "improve the delivery of healthcare services" [5] and especially "to improve emergency care in low- and middle-income countries" [7]. However, the global healthcare system is keeping used analog (paper-based) medical records, especially that this is the order in the majority of healthcare systems of low- and middle-income countries [6–8], while the healthcare systems in the high-income countries are slowly adopting the digital medical record systems [5, 6].

According to the "The Free Dictionary," emergency medical care (EMC) is defined as *providing life-saving measures in life-threatening situations*. Schneider et al. had defined the emergency medical care as "Emergency Medicine is the medical specialty with the principal mission of evaluating, managing, treating and preventing unexpected illness and injury" [9]. Riner, a medical doctor (MD)/emergency physician (EP) defined in 2011 in a post the emergency medical care as "the sudden onset of a medical condition manifesting itself by acute symptoms of sufficient severity (including server pain) such that the absence of immediate medical attention could reasonably be expected to result in: placing the patient's health in serious jeopardy, serious impairment to bodily functions, or serious dysfunction of any bodily organ or part." [10]. According to Riner, life-saving care must timely be provided. Time is then an important factor in the emergency medical care.

The common generic scenario in MEC is to transport an injured person from an accident place to the emergency services (commonly called emergency room) at a hospital, where he will be intensively treated. The emergency doctor in charge to transport the injured person to the close emergency care center is requested to stabilize him in providing life-saving first treatment during the transport. The emergency doctor (ED) needs patient-centric information for the primary care during the transport and has to timely provide the emergency center with the collected data and information about provided treatment and his diagnostics. Diagnostics made remotely based on patient-centered information provided through the emergency call need to be confirmed or revised once the injured person reaches the emergency center or the ED arrives at the accident place. As Schneider et al. stated in [9], a patient at an emergency room gets screened to confirm or revise the first diagnostics:

> *"…The first contact with nursing staff and the EP during the screening examination in the ED confirms or modifies this initial determination. EPs are specifically trained in the rapid assessment and triage of all patient presentations regardless of patient age or gender. The EP's role is to organize and manage the emergency care system based in the ED."* [9].

Beyond this, the EP is considered as the manager with the mission to evaluate the life-threatening situation that the patient is facing. These operations request accurate data that are in the best case patient-centric and patient-centered. Accessing these data can be time-consuming; therefore, the EP and whole nursing staff need to be assisted by modern technologies to gain time and quickly efficiently provide the first life-saving care to the patient within the golden hour. The golden time, critical where one can lose the injured, is the first hour between the accident occurs and the time the injured receives the first aid. In certain cases, the golden hour is less than 60 min. In this golden time, the emergency has to prevent the injured from any life-threatening medical issues.

Modern information and communication and data security technologies can contribute to collect, process, and store important data and quickly retrieve these data in the case of emergency as well as assure data security. Wireless sensor networks (WSNs) especially the wireless body area network (WBAN) are technologies that can help to collect and ensure data.

The chapter presents a concept for improving emergency medical care process and services delivery in the developing countries. It further pursues the objectives to connect the unconnected health things to enable patient-centric emergency medical care delivery using the Internet of Things paradigm. Data security, communication protocols, and technologies are out of the scope of this chapter. There are various previous works such as [11] that have already covered the EHR access control.

The remainder of this chapter is structured as follows: (i) Section 2 presents the state of the art (literature review) regarding the usage of the Internet of Things in medical application and especially in the emergency medical care. The research objectives and context are presented in Section 3. The technical background is briefly presented in Section 4. The concept and architecture are described in Section 5. The proof of concept (experiment) is presented in Section 6. The test results are discussed in Section 7. Section 8 concludes the chapter.

2. Related works

This section provides a short but comprehensive literature review on the use of the Internet of Things in medical applications like remote medical monitoring using various modern technologies such the wireless technology. It further investigates the state of the art on the use of the Internet of Things in delivering emergency medical care and the patient-centric medical care delivery.

2.1. Wireless sensor network in medical applications

The wireless sensor networks (WSNs) are being used by the healthcare industries to measure patient's vital parameter through medical sensors that are attached to his body. Bio-signals like body temperature, blood pressure, pulse oximetry, ECG, and breathing activity are, thus, sensed. Further, remote medical centers use end-point devices like video and audio devices to perform advance patient's monitoring [12].

In a multi-tier WSN, tasks are assigned to different nodes, where certain nodes (e.g., sensors) are assigned to simple tasks with low energy consumption. Low energy consuming nodes last for a long time and best fit for sensing data in healthcare applications. Multi-tier architectures have been used in similar applications like SensEye [13] and IrisNet [14] and have proven to be efficient. Moghadam et al. develop in [15] "an energy efficient data transmission technique for communication between a single-antenna medical sensor/microrobot inside the body to multi-antenna receiver on the body surface though non-homogeneous propagation environment."

Sensing data from the human body and transmitting over multiple spatial and temporal scales remain the first critical challenges in advanced health informatics [16]. In [17, 18] a noninvasive in vivo glucose sensors for measuring the blood glucose level was developed. In [19], the authors proposed a platform that combines IoT end-point devices (e. g. wearable sensors) with in-home healthcare services to improve user experience and service efficiency.

M. Mazhar Rathore et al. have discussed the presence of the Internet of Things in the medical sector and the amount of data these systems produce [20]. The wireless body area network (WBAN), a subset of the wireless sensor networks (WSNs), is using in the healthcare's applications to monitor the patient bio-signal [21].

In a previous article, the author presents a wireless sensor network system used at a cardiologic intensive care unit (CICU) to monitor the cardiologic in-patient and the ambient air in the hospital rooms. The patients are attached to a WSN that collect in real time the patients' vital parameters [22]. The experiment described in [22] has demonstrated that the WSN systems show a promise in collecting and retrieving medical data.

2.2. Internet of Things in the emergency medical care

The Internet of Things (IoT) especially the Internet of Health Things (IoHT) presents various potentialities for enhancing the emergency medical care from the beginning of the process till to the admission of the patient at the emergency room.

The emergency operation begins with the first call at the emergency coordination station. At this stage, the call center personal collects under time pressure important information on the occurrence. Most callers are, however, not able to correctly report the event and give information about the exact place of the event. In [23] the contributors proposed an IoT-based smart technology that can overcome the challenges facing the emergency call by automatically provide additional data. The data could be embedded the patient data in the emergency call. Such a system will enhance the emergency response and save time as well as reduce the death rate. In [24], the authors present a comprehensive survey on the usage of IoT in the medical field. Systems to handle the emergency medical care regarding the use of semantics and ontologies in sharing a large amount of medical data as well as data analysis have been described. The survey also presents the so-called indirect emergency health care that aims to assure data availability. Data availability requires data collection at a previous stage. This can happen through the medical record. The survey further discusses a medical record system that enables remote medical advice. It recommends reading the given paper to get more insight into the state of the art on the use of IoT in the health care.

The IoT is facing various challenges such as interoperability, security, authenticity, etc., because of the diversity of objects that can be involved in an IoT system as well as the size of the network that can issue security challenges. In [24], the authors present in an experiment a concept to meet the interoperability challenges in IoT systems. Interoperability can represent a barrier and especially an important issue in the emergency care. IoT system for emergency cases in China is presented in [25]. The authors describe an IoT-based system to monitor blood donation. This system can also help to set personal medical files. A remote monitoring and management platform of healthcare information, similar to that described in [22], is described in [26]. This system shows the potential of using the WSNs (IoT) in the health care. Various advantages of using IoT in the health care are described in [27]. The authors present an interesting aspect "The Anti-counterfeit of Medical Equipment and Medication."

As discussed earlier, the emergency response phase is an important phase of the whole process. Errors occurred at this phase can be hardly corrected. It is, therefore, important to avoid errors at this phase. In [28], the authors pose two research hypotheses as follows: (i) *H1: IoT technology fits the identified information requirements* and (ii) *H2: IoT technology provides added value to emergency response operations in terms of obtaining efficient cooperation, accurate situational awareness, and complete visibility of resources.*

Their findings fit the hypotheses and thus show that using IoT at emergency calling and response processing can enhance the emergency care.

2.3. Patient-centric and patient-centered emergency care delivery

2.3.1. Brief definition

Patient centricity: Patient-centric information is the information that emanates from the patient himself added to the data that are mined from the (electronic) medical and/or health records, which in turn must include genomic information, which enables to detect any disease predisposition [29].

Patient-centered care: Patient-centered care is a visit-based care, which means that patient-centered information is the information the patient and/or his parents provide the physician with [30].

2.3.2. Patient-centric versus patient-centered information

The patient-centered information originates from the patient and is mostly concerning the patient's needs and preferences regarding his healthcare concerns. It relies on the communication and a good relationship between the patient, patient's relatives, and the treating personnel. Starfield points out in [30] that patient-centered information or care rests on core elements such as communication or interaction and adherence to the recommendation concerning the care. It is determined by the interaction between patient and medical doctors [31].

The patient-centric information is directly produced by the patient himself added to the data that are mined from the (electronic) medical and/or health records, which in turn must include genomic information, which enables to figure out any disease predisposition.

The modern wireless technologies are used to collect the patient vital parameters as well as to filter clinical document to gain patient-centric data. The use of patient-centric information including genomic data in the emergency care is still not in order. Medical records do not include genomic information yet [32], and only few healthcare professionals are using electronic medical and/or health records [6].

2.3.3. Usage of patient-centric information in medical care

The use of electronic health records (EHR) in the medical care delivery impacts positively the treatment outcomes [31, 32]. In [33] the authors have shown that context-aware data and patient-centric decision-making are vital for personalized healthcare delivery. They discuss the challenges facing these new paradigms in wirelessly collecting physiological data and consequently proposed patient-centric care delivery for ubiquitous health care. The study found out that the proposed patient-centric information "will significantly improve the response time, quality, and relevance of data- and compute-intensive medical applications."

To our best knowledge, patient-centric-based emergency care delivery is still at an embryonic stage. The comprehensive literature review has shown that only few research works have been done regarding the topic. However, the terms are often mixed up or confused. Earlier articles written on the topic have confused patient-centric with patient-centered information. In [34] one can note this regarding the definition the authors made. This can be the reason why only a few articles handle the topic.

3. Objectives, context, and ethical approval

The main objective pursued in this study is to enhance the emergency medical care process from the response operation till to the hospital admission, especially in the developing countries, using IoT to autonomously and automatically provide in real time the emergency healthcare professionals and the emergency care centers with accurate and appropriate patient-centric information and, thus, substantially reduce the death rate.

This study aims at enhancing the data provision and exchange for a data-driven, patient-centric, and patient-centered emergency care.

At the present stage, the study focuses on the improvement of the emergency process in the case of a road accident in the developing countries. The developing countries and the road traffic injury represent therefore the research context of the study. The main reason for this choice is (i) the several healthcare access issues people are facing, (ii) the challenges the emergency transportation is facing, (iii) the lack of information and communications technology infrastructure, and the information paucity in the medical sector. The developed countries will also be considered. For evaluation purposes, cohorts of participants were built to simulate, test, and evaluate the different systems proposed. In collaboration with involved clinics and hospitals, we recruit patients using snowball approach. Each involved individual gives his consent so that their data can be collected, processed, and stored. The data were anonymously collected, processed, and stored. We also apply for ethical approval at the involved hospitals and clinics as well as at local municipal authorities.

4. Technical background

4.1. Internet of Health Things (IoHT)

Internet of Health Things (IoHT) integrates health objects with network connectivity from the digital and physical world. Furthermore, it combines personal health technologies and IoT and takes full advantages of IoT in expanding abilities to exchange useful data and enable improvements in context awareness and the ability to initiate actions based on data that are collected and analyzed [35].

4.2. Device-to-device (D2D) communication

Device-to-device (D2D) communication enables devices to communicate directly without interaction of base stations or access point. It is intended to exchange data utilizing various technologies such as ultrawideband (UWB), near-field communications (NFC), Zigbee, Bluetooth, Wi-Fi Direct, or LTE Direct. The distance between the devices is relatively short and defined by the using protocol. The communication is technology dependent [36].

4.3. Machine-to-machine (M2M) communication

M2M is an autonomous communication, based on a cellular network such as GSM, LTE, etc., where the communication passes through core networks via base stations or access points and M2M Server (application server). Compared with D2D, the communication is not direct and does not matter if the devices are approximate to one other. The distance between the devices is unlimited. Furthermore, the M2M communication is application oriented and technology independent (interoperability) [36].

4.4. Wireless sensor network (WSN)

WSN refers to a group of spatially dispersed and dedicated sensors for monitoring and recording the physical conditions of the environment and organizing the collected data at a central location. Sensors, within the network, sense and process data and communicate with each other [7]. WSNs are intended for efficient and cost-effective medical monitoring/surveillance for deployment at emergency medical care centers so that health professionals can easily monitor their in-patients irrespective of location and time and thus collect important bio-signals and environmental data for an effective treatment.

4.5. Crowdsensing

Crowdsensing is a critical component of the Internet of Things [37]. Crowdsourced data can be collected using participatory or opportunistic crowdsensing paradigms, where participants' smartphone sensors are used to collect information/data. Smartphone sensors or sensor systems are increasingly used for measuring the quality of ambient air [38] and temperature and particularly sensing bio-signals within an in- or outdoor crowd.

4.5.1. Participatory versus opportunistic sensing

Crowdsensing systems are either participatory or opportunistic. Participatory crowdsensing requires participants' active involvement: participants perform computations and generate data as inputs for the systems, while in opportunistic crowdsensing requires fewer participants' involvement: sensing is more autonomous, data are automatically generated without user involvement, and computations are also automatically performed using participants' devices or available sensors [39].

5. IoT-enabled emergency medical care services delivery

This section describes the proposed IoT-based patient-centric information processing system for improving the global emergency medical care services delivery and especially equipping the developing countries' emergency medical care systems with an adapted and context-sensitive emergency medical care system.

A distributed and federated medical record that includes information like genomic information as designed and implemented in [6] is the central piece of the proposed patient-centric information system that uses the IoT paradigm to collect, store, and process data. The EMR is accessible to any emergency doctor during an emergency transportation. The EMR features components like emergency cases relating to information, medical case files, and genomic files including disease predisposition information.

Additionally, a crowdsensing-based road traffic congestion detection unit is featured and contributes to early detect road traffic congestion and consequently compute an alternative route to quickly attend the emergency center closer to the accident place.

The emergency calling disposes an IoT-based calling system capable to embed the injured person's emergency data, data of place of the occurrence, geographical data, and personal data of the caller in emergency response that will be forwarded to emergency doctor and emergency transportation unit.

Wireless sensor network technology is used to collect patient-centric data and timely update the EMR. Furthermore, the proposed should enable to autonomously, automatically, and contactlessly exchange data with the information desk at the emergency care hospital and any computer networking wireless devices that can ad hoc be registered and connected to the ambulatory emergency care information system for providing or collecting data.

The communication between the proposed system and the information desk as well as any wireless (mobile) devices will follow the D2D and/or M2M communication paradigms. The communication within the system is based on M2M communication paradigm to prevent the interoperability issues and to enable the machines (physical or logical) to use different communication technologies and protocols to easily communicate with each other.

5.1. Crowdsensing-based road congestion detection

The emergency transportation system in the most developing countries is inadequate. The road traffic net is in a bad state, and medical helicopter does not exist. A real-time road traffic congestion detection is, therefore, so important to prevent any delay in emergency transportation. Developed countries also face road congestion at the pick hours or by an accident event. The proposed crowdsensing-based road traffic congestion detection system can be adapted and thus used in the developed countries too (reverse innovation). Over the past years, many efforts in monitoring the road traffic to prevent road traffic congestion and accident are done. The IoT vehicle-to-vehicle (V2V) technology is used to implement such systems. Various research works were and are still being conducted on the topic (see [40–46]). Implementing such system in the developing countries is easier than in the developed countries since personal data protection or data privacy act is less restrictive in the developing world. Alternative solution approaches based on inter-vehicular communication with respect to the data privacy and security have been discussed in [42, 47].

The proposed congestion detection system takes into account the technological level, the ICT, and municipal infrastructure available in the developing world. Technologies like inter-vehicular communication, vehicle-to-vehicle (V2V) communication, infrastructure-to-infrastructure (I2I) communication are not implementable in these countries, though crowdsensing paradigm can be implemented since smartphones with embedded cameras are available and the regions are well covered by mobile telecommunication infrastructure. The requirements for a standard crowdsensing are met here, and thus the proposed road traffic congestion detection system can be implemented here. The system aims at combining both participatory and real-time opportunistic crowdsensing and crowdsourcing data to energy-efficiently and low-cost monitor ad hoc traffic crowds for early detection of traffic jam risks.

A cloud-based algorithm requests continuously participant's mobile phone on given routes to provide information on the traffic. These participants are requested to activate the client application installed on their mobile phones to participate in the traffic monitoring. The client application measures the density of the traffic in reporting their GSP coordinates to the cloud. The client could recognize which GSP coordinates are useful for detecting a traffic congestion.

The proposed detection system aims at detecting the congestion at a crossroad as well as measure the congestion length. Each traffic light has GSP coordinates. The detection's algorithm monitors every activity within 2 kilometers around the traffic light using all smartphone coordinates in this circle. Thus, the speed of each vehicle or motorcycle on the given route can be determined, and, thus, traffic jam can be detected if it occurs. Similar work has been conducted and presented in [42] where the authors use the vehicle-to-vehicle paradigm to detect traffic congestion. Li Wei et al. propose in [48] a real-time road congestion detection in estimating vehicle density based on texture analysis and evaluate the system. The results demonstrate the potentiality of this approach.

As Zhu et al. in [49], the traffic is categorized, after an observational study, in peak and flat period. From 10 pm to 4 am the next day, we have a flat traffic. From 5 am to 9 am, the road congestion is high as well as the accident risk. Between 7 pm and 9 pm, road congestion can again be noted. The algorithm considers all this information in searching the appropriate route. This algorithm also uses the travel salesman algorithm in calculating the route for a quick transportation of the patient from the accident place to the next hospital. In [50] a model to optimize a network traffic flow is proposed. The model can be implemented to enable low-delay vehicular traffic flow. The proposed model shows a promise for low-delay vehicular traffic flow control from which emergency transportation can take benefit.

5.2. Federated electronic medical records (fEMR)

The patient medical record (MR) includes emergency data and medical case files and is a central piece of the concept. The clinical documentation (CD) is a digital or analog record tracking all medical treatment and related activities. MR and CD are part of the hospital information system (HIS). The clinical documentation serves as the basis and benchmark medical information document for further medical activities (e.g., treatment) or investigation on prior treatment; therefore, it must be accurate, must be timely filled, and must prevent any data privacy issues. It further can serve to create complete patient medical records including medical data from different medical institutions.

A hospital information system (HIS) must ensure that the patient medical and health records, as well as the clinical documentation, are always available, reliable, and data privacy assured. Available medical record at anytime and anywhere is an important piece in efficient, effective, and timely emergency care services delivery; beyond the availability aspect, the accuracy and the authenticity of the information/data contained in such document are very important for any further medical activities. The medical record must be up to date and well written (in the case the practitioner likes to write a medical assessment into the record).

The proposed MR (**Figure 1**) is a federated electronic MR (fEMR) equivalent to an electronic health record (EHR). It lies on a federated database system (FDB) and collects patient's medical records from all available sources. The so collected data is stored in the central database. An algorithm performs autonomously and automatically this job one to two times a day. An FDB is "a federated database system is a collection of independent, autonomous database systems, each with their own set of global users, which cooperate together to form an alliance or federation that enables global users to access data across the participating systems in a transparent manner." [51].

The fEMR can be connected to WSNs designed and implemented for collecting data within an emergency transportation. Once the emergency call is completed and all needed information is collected, the call center assigns an ambulance and an emergency doctor to the case. The patient's fEMR is connected to the WSN system in the ambulance. The patient-centric information is then set and can start collecting data emanating from the patient and automatically update the EMR. Accident report unit is featured by the EMR and is filled during the emergency calling phase. The emergency doctor (ED) can add more details to accident report once he is at the accident and collect patient-centered information.

The fEMR system can be used in on- and offline mode. Offline modus is considered for regions where the access to the Internet is limited or nonexistent. The ED can then download a lightweight version of the patient's fEMR and use it for his purposes. The data added newly to the local copy of the patient's fEMR will then be synchronized with the cloud-hosted fEMR if the Internet access is again available. A backend routine performs this task automatically.

5.2.1. Emergency data and medical case files

Patient emergency data (PED) are medical data that are necessary rather mandatory during the golden hours in the case of emergency. It is, for example, vital in a case of emergency to

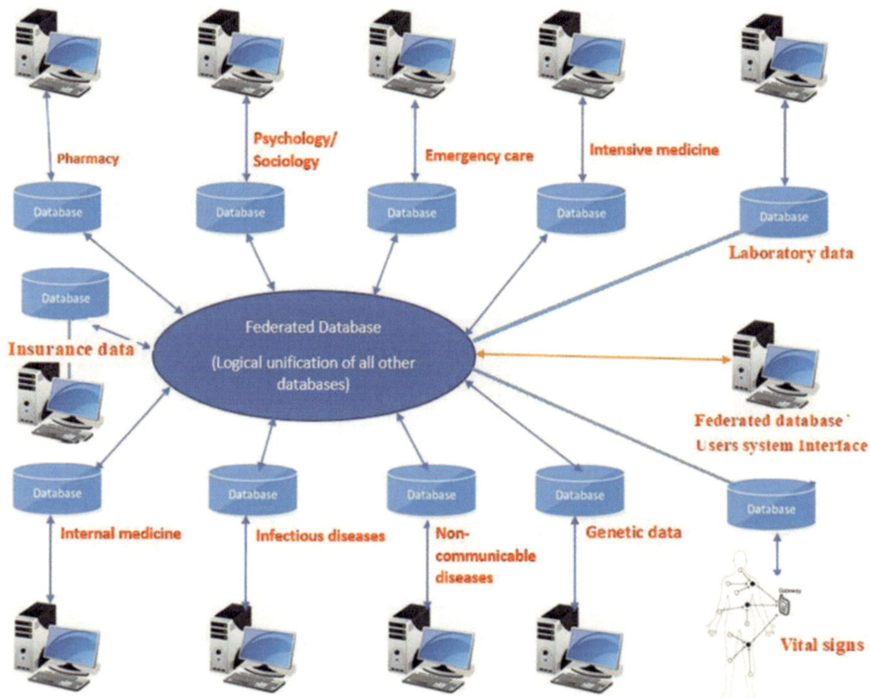

Figure 1. Architectural view of the proposed federated electronic medical records.

have accurate information on the diabetic condition of an individual or his serologic status or the list of his current medication to prevent any drug intoxication. The emergency data are created automatically set by the EMR system. Any treating physician can add emergency care-relevant information. The emergency data is stored on the patient's electronic health card as well as in the EMR in the central database.

The emergency data includes the allergies, the medicinal treatments, the medical risks, and the avoidable medical attacks, i.e., any procedures, which are life-threatening for the patient. These data are updated regularly and must be reliable. The emergency data must be always available.

The diagnostics or medical case file includes the picture of a specific illness, the treatments performed, and the course of the illness. This information is purposely created ad hoc to facilitate the decision-making regarding any medical activity concerning the patient.

5.3. Resulting architecture

5.3.1. Connecting the unconnected (emergency room, ambulance, and fEMR)

The architectural view of a standard patient-centric emergency care delivery is illustrated in **Figure 2**. The proposed standard patient-centric and IoT-based emergency care services delivery system combine collecting vital parameters (on the patient within the transportation) using WBAN/WSN technology with the retrieving health records from the fEMR. The system filters the needed data from these different sources and presents them to the medical doctor. The data collected through the WBAN are automatically processed and stored in the fEMR.

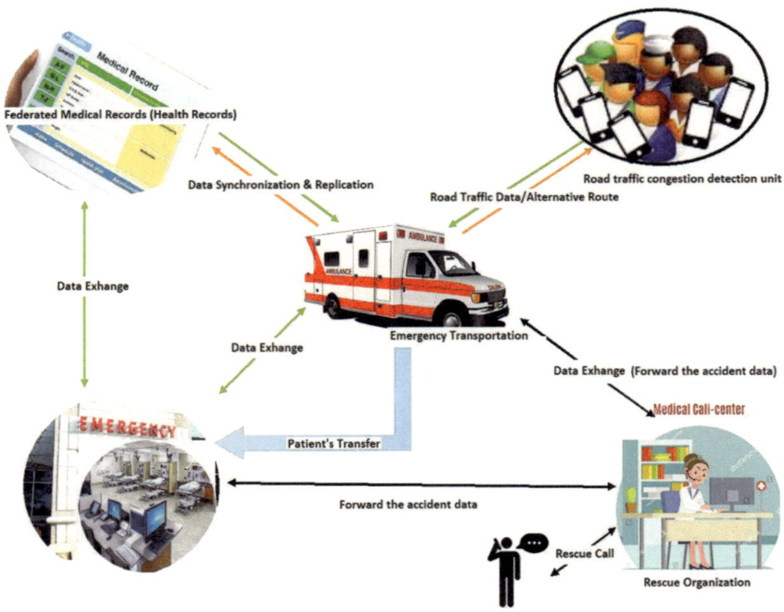

Figure 2. Standard patient-centric emergency care delivery process.

http://dx.doi.org/10.5772/intechopen.76974

The patient-centered data or information are recorded and stored in the fEMR. A voice-based interface oversees collecting audio information and stores it local and remote.

The call center is featured with an M2M-based system that autonomously embeds the accident data in the patient's fEMR, sends it automatically to the emergency transportation unit, and determines the geo-position of the accident.

A road traffic congestion unit contributes to finding the right routes to preventing road traffic congestion. This component is specially designed for developing counties since developed countries dispose of adequate road traffic monitoring systems and can use medical helicopters to emergency transportation. As earlier described, this component fits the road nets in the developing countries and is context-aware.

There exists an ICT infrastructure gap between the developing and developed countries [6]. The concept takes, therefore, an account for this fact and proposes an adapted patient-centric and IoT-based emergence care services delivery in the case of road traffic accident. At the rural level, emergency care transportation logistics are scarce or nonexistent. Often, it is very hard to quickly attend those areas due to the bad state of the road. To overcome this challenge, the near dispensary will request a nonmedical car and remotely instruct the driver as well as the rescue caller on how to transport the injured to the next dispensary. Each care is supposed to have a well-equipped pharmacy for the first aid on board. Car drivers are also supposed to be trained to give first aid. At the same time, an ambulance will be requested from the near emergency center. This operation has the potential to save time and provide the first aid to the injured. Imagine, healthcare professionals at a dispensary must go the accident scenes that can be several kilometers far away before the injured will receive the first aid. This scenario

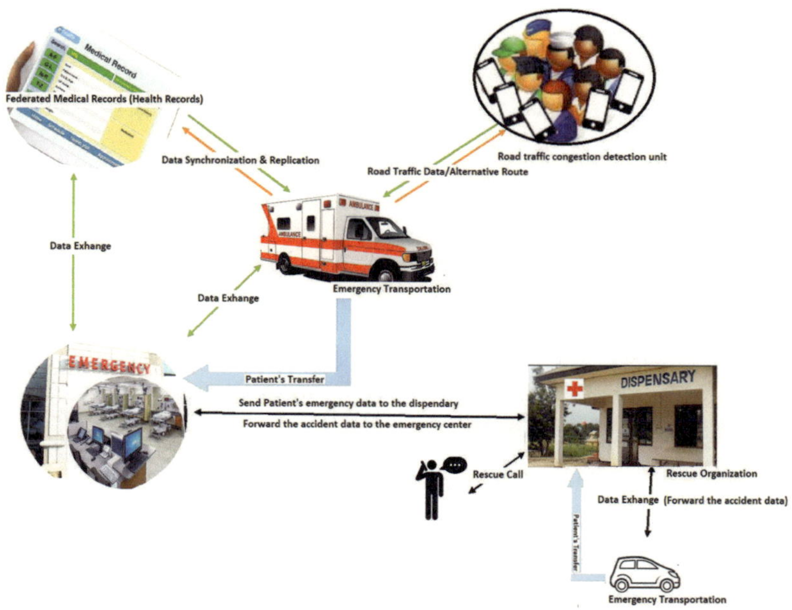

Figure 3. Patient-centric emergency care delivery process when the accident occurs in rural regions.

can lead to the injured death or cause him/her serious disability. To prevent such a situation, the dispensary personnel will remotely and accordingly instruct the relatives of the injured person with the information from the patient fEMR. The instructions are based on the patient-centric information. Once the injured person is delivered to the dispensary, an ambulance will transport him to the next emergency care center. **Figure 3** illustrates an emergency care delivery process at the rural level.

6. Experiment, methodology, and materials

This section will shortly present the conducted experiment, study methodology, and materials.

The global concept, as well as the appropriate architecture for improving the emergency care delivery, was tested at the rural level. A test cohort was built and an accident scene in a village was simulated. The area was selected according to following criteria: (i) lack of ambulance, (ii) very difficult road accessibility, (iii) the next dispensary is at 30 km, and (iv) mobile phone and telecommunication are possible.

Two car drivers, one with an approved medical first aid training and one without approved medical first aid training, and a less-educated caller are recruited. The reason why we select a less-educated call is to simulate the real situation, where the caller is often confused. The car driver without medical first aid training is selected to test the impact of the training on completing instructions received from a remote healthcare professional.

A dummy fEMR is generated. The accident scene is set up. Three data-driven emergency care delivery scenarios were simulated: (i) a patient-centric emergency care delivery, (ii) a patient-centered emergency care delivery, and (iii) emergency care delivery based on patient-centric combined with patient-centered information. **Table 1** indicates the test scenarios and outcomes with their characteristics. The impact of the first aid training on the care delivery is also investigated.

A rapid prototype of the proposed system was implemented. The server-side application was hosted on a GlassFish 4.0.1 on a laptop. A client application is used to visualize received data. The client application on the smartphone (gateway, sensors) communicates directly with the server application.

A qualitative data analysis is done using r-data analytics tool and following approaches: (i) organizing the data, (ii) identifying the framework, (iii) sorting the data into the framework, and (iv) using the framework for descriptive analysis.

The car driver with approved training in medical first aid successfully completed his assigned task in accordance with the instructions of the remote healthcare professional, and he has timely delivered the injured to the dispensary without additional damages. However, the other driver, without approved training in medical first aid, was less successful in completing his tasks despite the received instruction.

Test scenarios	Characteristics of the car driver		Origin of the information used	
	Approved training	No approved training	Patient-centric information	Patient-centered information
Test 1	x		x	
Test 2	x			x
Test 3		x	x	
Test 4		x		x
Test 5	x		x	x
Test 6		x	x	x

x means which information is used and what is the training level of the car driver involved. For example, Test 1 involves car driver with approved training and used data emanated from the patient (patient-centric information).

Table 1. Simulation scenarios for emergency medical care services delivery.

The experiment that uses patient-centric information has shown that beyond the standard emergency care, personalized care was provided through the information from the fEMR. The simulation with patient-centered information was also successful, but no personalized care was provided. Furthermore, the collected data within the emergency care were locally processed and archived at the emergency center and likely will not be used for further care provision. In contrary, data that were collected within the patient-centric emergency care provision are stored and processed in the cloud and the fEMR is synchronized and up to date. Information about the transportation duration, the quality of the primary care delivery, and the outcomes are collected.

The test's main objective was to figure out the impact of the medical first aid training on the outcomes and impact of the quality and source of the information on the outcomes.

7. Study results and discussions

7.1. Study limitation

Worst cases, where car drivers are not up to date regarding the medical first aid training (that means he was trained but forgets the essentials) or furthermore the case where nobody at the accident scene is trained to give medical first aid, are not tested.

The test period is relatively short. Furthermore, real emergency cases were not tested, and then such cases could provide more useful data for analysis.

7.2. Results and discussions

The car driver with approved training in medical first aid successfully completed his assigned task in accordance with the instructions of the remote healthcare professional, and he has timely delivered the injured to the dispensary without additional damages. However, the other driver, without approved training in medical first aid, was less successful in completing his tasks despite the received instruction.

The experiment that uses patient-centric information has shown that beyond the standard emergency care, personalized care was provided through the information from the fEMR. The simulation with patient-centered information was also successful, but no personalized care was provided. Furthermore, the collected data within the emergency care were locally processed and archived at the emergency center and likely will not be used for further care provision. In contrary, data that were collected within the patient-centric emergency care provision are stored and processed in the cloud and the fEMR is synchronized and up to date.

Reliability and validity: To ensure the reliability and validity of the test, each test scenario was repeated three times. The impact of the information used, as well as the training of the driver, was thus validated.

Accuracy of the collected data: Collected data must be accurate. Information about the golden hour, the collected bio-signal, and patient-provided information were valid.

Measurement errors rates: The error rates within the golden hour, in measuring bio-signal and in reporting the event at the hospital, were assessed. The error rate was negligible.

Impact of the training on the overall outcomes: The experiments have shown the impact of the training level on the overall outcome. It revealed the impact of the golden hour on the medical outcomes. Furthermore, tests involving trained drive have produced positive outcomes. The patient has high survival chance when, in addition to trained driver, nothing but patient-centric data is used, patient-centric combined with patient-centered data are used. The patient has less chances of survival when the driver is not trained and only patient-centered data is used.

Test	Outcomes
Test 1	Positive outcomes. The patient received adequate first aid due to the knowledge of the driver and the accurate patient-centric data available
Test 2	Negative outcomes. Information provided was incomplete (subject). This has negatively impacted the outcomes. The transportation was conservative, and then the driver knows how to prevent any additional medical or health damages
Test 3	Due to lack of first aid, the collected data could not be used in the golden hour. However, the patient received adequate care based on the collected data. The healthcare professionals have estimated that in real case the patient's chance to survive could be less than 40%, since he did not receive appropriate care in the golden hour and, additionally, the transportation was not conservative because the driver was not trained
Test 4	The outcome is similar to Test 3. However, the survival chance for the patient was estimated to 10%, and then the medical examinations were needed to verify the information provided by the patient
Test 5	Very positive outcome. All the needed information is available. The patient was stabilized in the golden hour. The transportation to the hospital was conservative. At the hospital, the patient received timely follow-up treatment (simulation). Timely because no medical treatment was needed. The patient-centric data is already available
Test 6	The outcomes are similar to those at Test 5. However, the transportation was not conservative, because the driver was not trained

Table 2. Test outcomes.

Table 2 summarizes the test outcomes.

8. Conclusion

Previous research works have demonstrated that health care is taking enormous benefit of the use of Internet of Things technology and paradigm in the healthcare provision. A comprehensive literature review has revealed that IoT technologies like WBAN and WSN are used for collecting, storing, and processing patient-centric data. The data processing takes a full benefit of the IoT technology, where data are autonomously and automatically collected. Fog/edge computing contributes to locally process with the collected data for quick decision-making. Quick decision-making is an important issue in the healthcare delivery regarding the time that is a critical point.

This study presents an IoT-enabled emergency medical care services delivery system working with patient-centric data (current and previously collected data) from different sources, including genomic data, which is not actually considered in medical treatment due to the high cost of genomic sequencing. The central piece of the proposed system is the federated electronic medical care that collects EMRs from different sources, adds the genomic part, and sets automatically the individual emergency care data as well as medical cases files on demand.

This system has presented a novelty. To our best knowledge, no emergency care system worldwide is using such a federated database like health record.

Conflict of interest

Author Edoh declares that he has no conflict of interest. Informed consent was obtained from all individual participants included in this study.

Author details

Thierry Edoh

Address all correspondence to: oscar.edoh@gmail.com

Technical University of Munich, Institut für Informatik/I1, München, Germany

References

[1] WHO. Global status report on Road Safety: Time for Action. Geneva: World Health Organization; 2009. Available from: www.who.int/violence_injury_prevention/road_safety_status/2009

[2] Macharia W, Njeru E, Muli-Musiime F, Nantulya V. Severe road traffic injuries in Kenya, quality of care and access. African Health Sciences. 2009;**9**(2):118-124

[3] Nicholson B, McCollough C, Wachira B, Mould-Millman NK. Emergency medical services (EMS) training in Kenya: Findings and recommendations from an educational assessment. African Journal of Emergency Medicine . 2017;**7**(4):157-159

[4] Razzak JA, Kellermann AL. Emergency medical care in developing countries: Is it worthwhile? Bulletin of the World Health Organization. 2002;**80**(11):900-905

[5] DesRoches CM, Campbell EG, Rao SR, Donelan K, Ferris TG, Jha A, Kaushal R, Levy DE, Rosenbaum S, Shields AE, Blumenthal D. Electronic health records in ambulatory care — A national survey of physicians. The New England Journal of Medicine. Jul 2008;**359**(1):50-60

[6] Edoh TOC. Advanced Systems for Improved Public Healthcare and Disease Prevention Emerging Research and Opportunities. USA: IGI Global, Medical Information Service Reference (an imprint of IGI Global). 2018

[7] Boonstra A, Broekhuis M. Barriers to the acceptance of electronic medical records by physicians from systematic review to taxonomy and interventions. BMC Health Services Research. 2010;**10**(231):1-17

[8] Edoh TO. ICT-Systeme zur Verbesserung der Gesundheitsversorgung in den Gesundheitssystemen der afrikanischen Entwicklungsländern. Fallstudien: Benin. Germany: Universität der Bundeswehr München: Athene-Forschung; 2010

[9] Schneider SM, Hamilton GC, Moyer P, Stapczynski JS. Definition of emergency medicine. Academic Emergency Medicine. June 2015;**5, 1998**:348-351

[10] Riner M (An emergency Physician). 2011. Available from: www.kevinmd.com [online]; https://www.kevinmd.com/blog/2011/11/definition-medical-emergency.html [Accessed: Jan 18, 2018]

[11] Charlotte UNC, Covington MJ, Hu H, Jin J, Ahn G-J, Zhang X. Patient-centric authorization framework for sharing electronic health records. In: ACM Digital Library, SACMAT '09 Proceedings of the 14th ACM symposium on Access Control Models and Technologies, Stresa, Italy. 2009. pp. 125-134

[12] Abed A, Alkhatib A, Baicher GS. Wireless sensor network architecture. International Conference on Computer Networks and Communication Systems. 2012;**35**(Cncs):11-15

[13] Kulkarni P, Ganesan D, Shenoy P, Lu Q. SensEye: A multi-tier camera sensor network. In: Multimedia '05 Proceedings of the 13th Annual ACM International Conference on Multimedia, Hilton, Singapore, 2005. No. February. pp. 229-238

[14] Campbell J, Gibbons P, Nath S, Pillai P, Seshan S, Sukthankar R. IrisNet: An internet-scale architecture for multimedia sensors. In: Proceedings of the 13th Annual ACM International Conference on Multimedia. ACM Digital Library; 2005. pp. 81-88

[15] Moghadam NN, Farhadi H, Bengtsson M. An energy efficient communication technique for medical implants/micro robots. In: Xplore IEEE 2016 10th International Symposium on Medical Information and Communication Technology (ISMICT). Xplore IEEE. 2016;**1**(1):1-5

[16] Yang G, Xie L, Mäntysalo M, Zhou X, Pang Z, Da Xu L, Kao-Walter S, Chen Q, Zheng LR. A health-IoT platform based on the integration of intelligent packaging, unobtrusive bio-sensor, and intelligent medicine box. IEEE Transactions on Industrial Informatics. 2014;**10**(4):2180-2191

[17] Bandodkar AJ, Jia W, Yardımcı C, Wang X, Ramirez J, Wang J. Tattoo-based noninvasive glucose monitoring: A proof-of-concept study. Analytical Chemistry. 2015;**87**(1):394-398

[18] Liakat S, Bors KA, Xu L, Woods CM, Doyle J, Gmachl CF. Noninvasive in vivo glucose sensing on human subjects using mid-infrared light. Biomedical Optics Express. 2014;**5**(7):2397

[19] On R, In E. Editorial note on the processing. Storage. 2010;**14**(4):895-896

[20] Rathore MM, Ahmad A, Paul A. The internet of things based medical emergency management using Hadoop ecosystem. In: Xplore IEEE 2015 IEEE Sensors. 2015. pp. 1-4

[21] Wan J, Zou C, Ullah S, Lai C-F, Zhou M, Wang X. Cloud-enabled wireless body area networks for pervasive healthcare. IEEE Network. 2013;**27**(5):56-61

[22] Edoh TOC, Atchome A, Alahassa BRU, Pawar P. Evaluation of a multi-tier heterogeneous sensor network for patient monitoring – The case of Benin. In: MMHealth '16 Proceedings of the 2016 ACM Workshop on Multimedia for Personal Health and Health Care. ACM Digital Library; 2016. pp. 23-29

[23] Bornheim M, Fletcher M, Al E. Public Safety Digital Transformation the Internet of Things (IoT) and Emergency Services. In: EENA Operations Document IoT and Emergency Services. 2016. pp. 1-26

[24] Riazul Islam SM, Kwak D, Humaun Kabir M, Hossain M, Kwak K-S. The internet of things for health care: A comprehensive survey. IEEE Access. 2015;**3**:678-708

[25] Ji Z, Anwen Q. The application of internet of things (IOT) in emergency management system in China. In: Xplore IEEE – 2010 IEEE Int. Conf. Technol. Homel. Secur. Xplore IEEE; 2010. pp. 139-142

[26] Zhao W, Wang C, Nakahira Y. Medical application on internet of things. In: IET Conf. Publ. IET Int. Conf. Commun. Technol. Appl. ICCTA 2011 Elsevier, vol. 2011, no. 586 CP, 2012. pp. 660-665

[27] Hu F, Xie D, Shen S. On the application of the internet of things in the field of medical and health care In: Proc. – 2013 IEEE Int. Conf. Green Comput. Commun. IEEE Internet Things IEEE Cyber, Phys. Soc. Comput. GreenCom-iThings-CPSCom. Xplore IEEE; 2013. pp. 2053-2058

[28] Yang L, Yang SH, Plotnick L. How the internet of things technology enhances emergency response operations. Technological Forecasting and Social Change. 2013;**80**(9):1854-1867

[29] Sheer DL. How Patient-Centric Care Differs from Patient-Centered Care. 2012. [Online]. Available from: https://davidleescher.wordpress.com/2012/03/03/how-patient-centric-care-differs-from-patient-centered-care-2/

[30] Starfield B. Is patient-centered care the same as person-focused care? The Permanente Journal. 2011;**15**(2):63-69

[31] Epstein RM, Fiscella K, Lesser CS, Stange KC. Analysis & commentary: Why the nation needs a policy push on patient-centered health care. Health Affairs. 2010;**29**(8):1489-1495

[32] Bates DW, Bitton A. The future of health information technology in the patient-centered medical home. Health Affairs. 2010;**29**(4):614-621

[33] Viswanathan H, Baozhi C, Pompili D. Research challenges in computation, communication, and context awareness for ubiquitous healthcare. IEEE Communications Magazine. 2012;**50**(5):92-99

[34] Barua M, Liang X, Lu R, Shen X. ESPAC: Enabling security and patient-centric access control for eHealth in cloud computing. International Journal of Security and Networks. 2011;**6**(2/3):67

[35] Terry N. Will the internet of health things disrupt healthcare? SSRN Electronic Journal. 2016;**19**(2):28-31

[36] Haus M, Waqas M, Ding AY, Li Y, Member S. Security and privacy in device-to-device (D2D) communication: A review. IEEE Communications Surveys & Tutorials. 2016;**19**(2):1054-1079

[37] Liu J, Shen H, Zhang X. A survey of mobile crowdsensing techniques: A critical component for the internet of things. In: 2016 25th International Conference on Computer Communication and Networks (ICCCN) Waikoloa, HI, USA, 2016

[38] Dutta J, Gazi F, Roy S, Chowdhury C. AirSense: Opportunistic crowd-sensing based air quality monitoring system for smart city. In: Xplore IEEE 2015 Ieee Sensors. 2016. pp. 1-3

[39] Chatzimilioudis G, Konstantinidis A, Laoudias C, Zeinalipour-yazti D. Crowdsourcing with smartphones. IEEE Internet Computing - IEEE Computer Society. 2012:1-7

[40] Martuscelli G, Boukerche A, Foschini L, Bellavista P. V2V protocols for traffic congestion discovery along routes of interest in VANETs: A quantitative study. Wireless Communications and Mobile Computing. Dec 2016;**16**(17):2907-2923

[41] Kirthiga N, Karthik S. Vehicular traffic re-routing for avoid the traffic congestion in VANET. International Journal of Innovative Research in Science Engineering and Technology. 2014;**3**(1):1530-1533

[42] Cárdenas-Benítez N, Aquino-Santos R, Magaña-Espinoza P, Aguilar-Velazco J, Edwards-Block A, Cass AM. Traffic congestion detection system through connected vehicles and big data. Sensors (Switzerland). 2016;**16**(5):1-26

[43] Milojevic M, Rakocevic V. Distributed road traffic congestion quantification using cooperative VANETs. In: 2014 13th Annu. Mediterr. Ad Hoc Netw. Work. Xplore IEEE 2013 IEEE Veh. Netw. Conf; 2014. pp. 203-210

[44] Jawhar I, Mohamed N, Usmani H. An overview of inter-vehicular communication systems, protocols and middleware. Journal of Networks. 2013;**8**(12):2749-2761

[45] Wang C, Tsai H-M. Detecting Urban Traffic Congestion with Single Vehicle. IEEE. 2013. pp. 233-240

[46] Milojevic M, Rakocevic V. Short paper: Distributed vehicular traffic congestion detection algorithm for urban environments. In: 2013 IEEE Veh. Netw. Conf. Xplore IEEE 2014 13th Annual Mediterranean Ad Hoc Networking Workshop (MED-HOC-NET); 2013. pp. 182-185

[47] Bauza R, Gozalvez J, Sanchez-Soriano J. Road traffic congestion detection through cooperative vehicle-to-vehicle communications. In: Proceedings - Conference on Local Computer Networks, (LCN), Denver, CO, USA; 2010. pp. 606-612

[48] Wei L, Dai H-Y. Real-time road congestion detection based on image texture analysis. Procedia Engineering. 2016;**137**:196-201

[49] Zhu Y, Gao N, Wang J, Liu C. Study on traffic flow patterns identification of single intersection intelligent signal control. Procedia Engineering. 2016;**137**:452-460

[50] Csikós A, Charalambous T, Farhadi H, Kulcsár B, Wymeersch H. Network traffic flow optimization under performance constraints. Transportation Research Part C: Emerging Technologies. 2017;**83**:120-133

[51] Grimson J, Grimson W, Berry D, Stephens G, Felton E, Kalra D, Toussaint P, Weier OW. A CORBA-based integration of distributed electronic healthcare records using the synapses approach. IEEE Transactions on Information Technology in Biomedicine. 1998;**2**(3):124-138

Chapter 2

Investigations of MIMO Antenna for Smart Mobile Handsets and Their User Proximity

Hari Shankar Singh

Additional information is available at the end of the chapter

http://dx.doi.org/10.5772/intechopen.75002

Abstract

In this chapter, a monopole antenna with compact size, simple structure, easy to fabricate is reported which covers LTE700 (band13/14) (746–798 MHz), GSM1800 (1710–1885 MHz), PCS1900 (1850–1990 MHz), and LTE2600 (2500–2690 MHz) band based on 6-dB return loss. The proposed MIMO antenna consists of two radiating elements. The main radiating element is a composition of driven element, which is directly fed with microstrip line, and one parasitic element. The parasitic element provides the resonance at higher frequency band and the combination of driven elements and parasitic elements provide above-said frequency bands. The current distribution, far-field radiation patterns, and diversity parameters are checked out for the MIMO antenna in free space. Further performances are studied in the presence of user proximity.

Keywords: diversity antenna, planar antenna, mobile phone, user proximity

1. Introduction

The fourth generation and Wi-MAX technologies require high data rates and longer range so that the end users can enjoy the quality service. In order to accomplish this, wireless communication systems have to be pushed to the physical limits of the radio channels [1]. As "a key to gigabit wireless" multiple-input multiple-output (MIMO) technology as a diversity scheme made a great breakthrough for raising the performance with high-speed transmission rates, high-quality mobile communication services without the need of any additional frequency spectrum or power [2, 3]. The vast potential of MIMO techniques is manifested by rapid espousal into the wireless standards, such as LTE (Long Term Evolution), UMTS, and Wi-MAX [4–7].

LTE standard is used for high speed and better quality communication of mobile phones and data terminals that can integrate MIMO technologies for reducing fading phenomenon, increasing channel capacity, and could be incorporated into handheld mobile applications [8, 9]. The most challenging task in MIMO systems is to enforce multiple antennas on handheld terminals as small as mobile handsets. Now-a-days, the slimness of mobile phone has been tremendously increased therefore, to keeping the volume of an antenna small, became a difficult task. The antennas are required to be small, designed with in the small volume and yet their functioning has to be maintained to achieve high gain, wide bandwidth, and low correlation coefficient. The use of inductors and capacitors are, to match of the resonance frequency, tuning of the frequency bands, and to increase the electrical length, but simultaneously reduces the bandwidth and the efficiency of the antenna due to these chip elements. Some of the literature available to make antenna electrically small size, and to obtain wider impedance bandwidth [10, 11]. A dual electrically small MIMO antenna system for 4G terminals was presented by Sharawi et al. which covered the band of 760–886 MHz [10]. Zhang et al. presented a wideband LTE MIMO antenna in mobile handset operating at 740 MHz [11]. The matching level and central frequency are tuned by the shunt capacitor of the port and the series inductor. Shen et al. introduce a wideband diversity antenna which operates in a very wide bandwidth of 1200 MHz starting from 1700 to 2900 MHz [12]. A compact Tri-band MIMO/diversity antenna for mobile was proposed which covers LTE band (765–787 MHz), PCS 1900 (1850–1920 MHz) and Wi-Max (3050–3650 MHz) [13]. The above-proposed antennas are complex in terms of fabrication (loaded with chip components like inductors and capacitors) and in design.

2. Antenna design and configuration

Figure 1(a) illustrates the specific geometry of the proposed antenna, consisting of two symmetrical back to back monopole antenna elements, which are printed on the upper corners of the mobile circuit board (FR4 substrate with $\varepsilon r = 4.4$ and $\tan \delta = 0.02$). The two antenna elements are considered in this study which are placed near to the corner of mobile phone. The dimension of the substrate is chosen as $120 \times 60 \times 0.8$ mm^3. On the upper surface of the substrate, the main rectangular ground of dimension 104×60 mm^2 is disposed. The volume of the single antenna element is $16 \times 21 \times 7$ mm^3 which are mounted at the top corner of the mobile circuit board. The enlarged view of the single unfolded antenna element is given **Figure 1(b)** whereas **Figure 1(c)** shows the detailed dimensions of the proposed slot configuration on the ground plane. Detailed dimensions of the unfolded metal strip are shown in **Figure 1(d)**. All optimized parameters are shown in **Table 1**.

http://dx.doi.org/10.5772/intechopen.75002

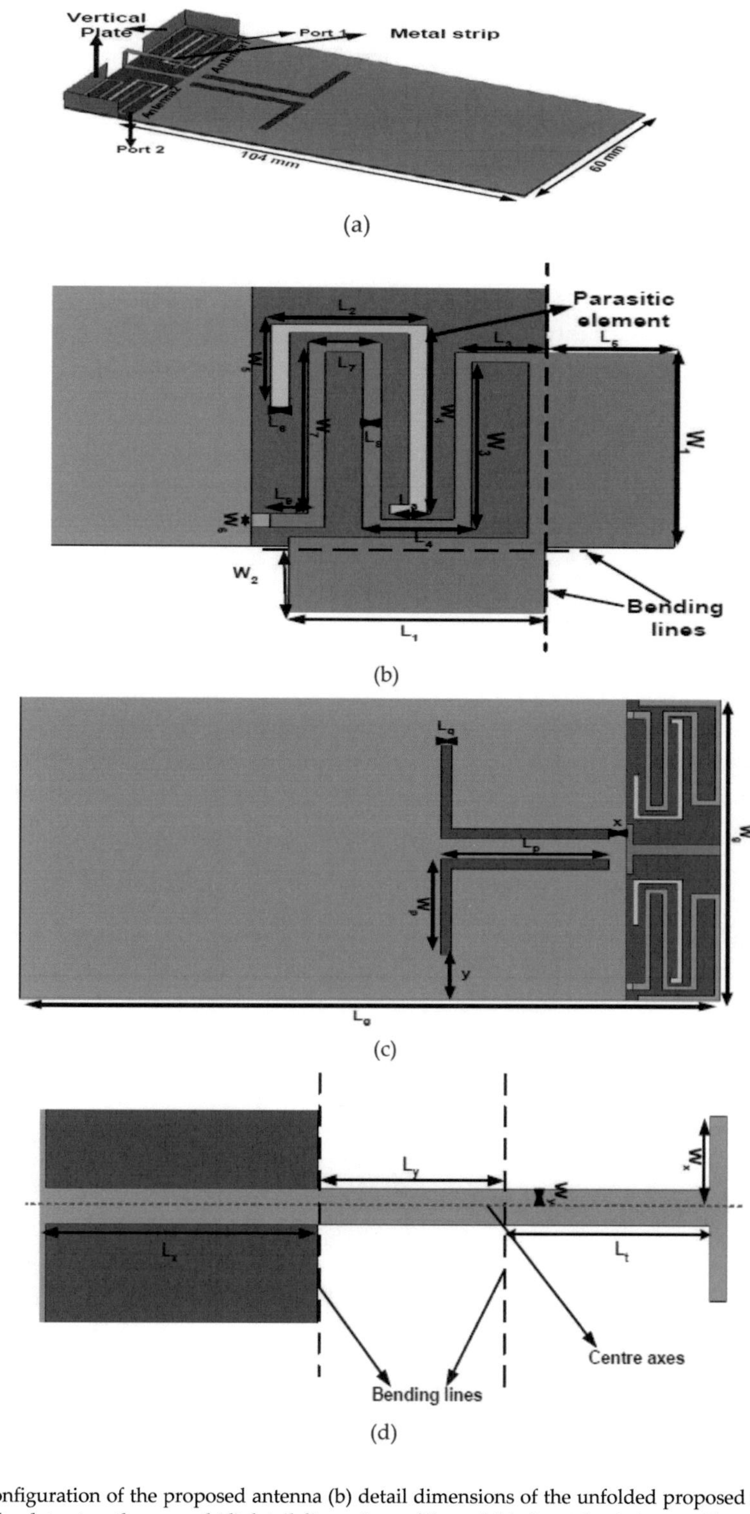

Figure 1. (a) Configuration of the proposed antenna (b) detail dimensions of the unfolded proposed antenna (c) detail dimensions of the slot cut on the ground (d) detail dimensions of the unfolded metal strip inserted between the antennas.

Parameter	Value (mm)	Parameter	Value (mm)	Parameter	Value (mm)
L_g	120	L_6	1	W_6	1.5
W_g	60	L_7	4	W_7	18.5
L_1	14	L_8	1	L_a	10
W_1	21	L_9	2	L_q	2
L_2	8.5	W_2	7	L_p	27
L_3	5	W_3	18	W_p	17
L_4	6	W_4	20.5	x	3
L_5	7	W_5	9	y	9
L_x	16	L_y	7	L_t	16
W_x	5	W_y	1		

Table 1. Optimized shape parameters of the proposed antenna.

3. Results and discussions

3.1. *S*-parameter analysis

All the simulations are carried out on finite element method (FEM) based high-frequency structure simulator (HFSS). **Figure 2** shows the optimized *S*11 and *S*21 parameters of the proposed antenna. The reported antenna covers operating band at lower frequency side from 736 to 822 MHz, and at higher frequency side from 1609 to 2057 MHz, and from 2491 to 2785 MHz based on the 6-dB return loss. Which covers the LTE700 (band13/14), GSM1800, PCS1900, and LTE2600 mobile communication bands. The achieve isolation between MIMO

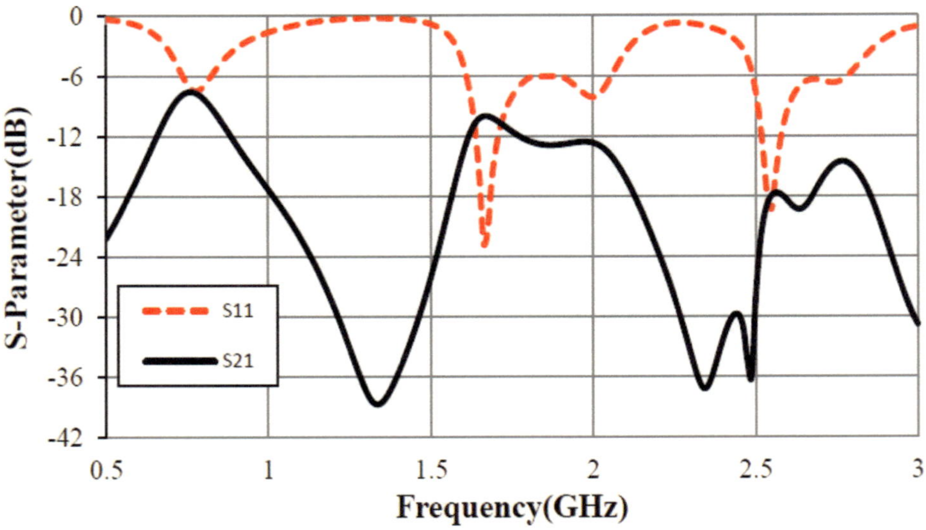

Figure 2. *S*-parameter of the proposed MIMO antenna.

http://dx.doi.org/10.5772/intechopen.75002

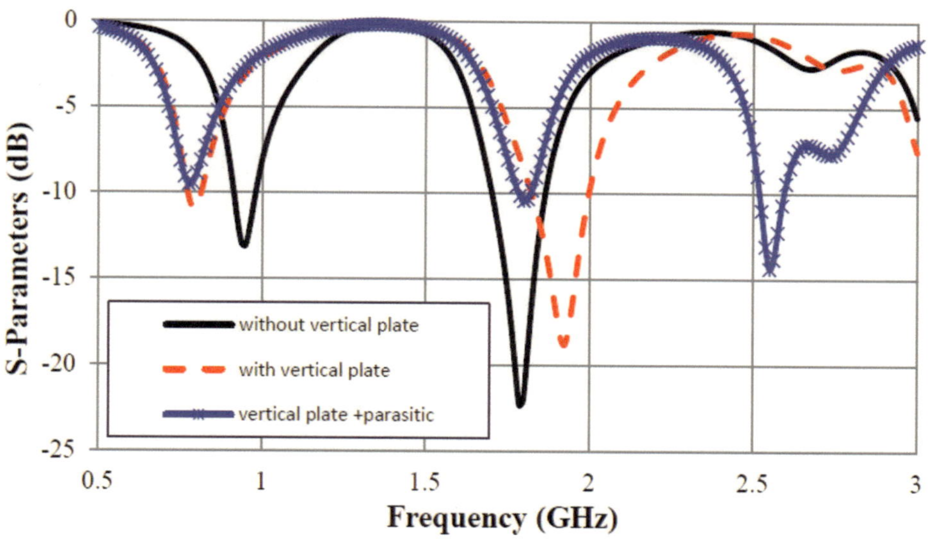

Figure 3. Effect of the vertical plate and the parasitic element on the *S*-parameters.

antenna elements are −7.5 dB across 775 MHz (736–822 MHz), −10 dB across 1660 MHz (1609–2057 MHz), and better than −18 dB over 2.55 GHz (2491–2785 MHz).

The main driven element which is directly fed by a microstrip line is designed to resonate at 937 MHz simultaneously higher modes provide another resonance centered at 1787 MHz. A parasitic element is used which resonates at 2.55 GHz. To achieve the LTE700 frequency band the vertical plate is added to the main radiating element due to which the electrical length is increased correspondingly the lower operating frequency is shifted from 937 to 762 MHz as shown in **Figure 3**.

3.2. Parametric analysis

Figure 4 shows the variation of *S*-parameters with different configurations. There are two different configurations analyze to see the effect on *S*-parameters. In the first configuration, only ground slot is present means no metal strip present between antenna elements, due to this modification the isolation is increased at higher frequency side whereas the isolation remains same at lower frequency side. When the only metal strip is present means no ground slot the bandwidth enhancement is observed. Further, these two modifications combined into single structure and variation of *S*-parameters is shown in **Figure 5**. It is observed that isolation, as well as bandwidth, gets enhanced by adding metal strip and slot on the ground.

Some key parameters are optimized for proper bandwidth and impedance matching at lower frequency side as well as higher frequency side. **Figure 6** shows the effect of 'W_1' on *S*-parameters. It is seen that as 'W_1' increase, bandwidth decreases at the middle band and bandwidth increases at the upper frequency whereas isolation over operating bands almost unaffected. The optimized value for 'W_1' is 21 mm. **Figure 7** shows the effect of the parameter 'W_x'. It is observed that as the value of 'W_x' increases, the isolation at 1.65 GHz, and at 2.54 GHz decreases. The optimized value of 'W_x' is 5 mm.

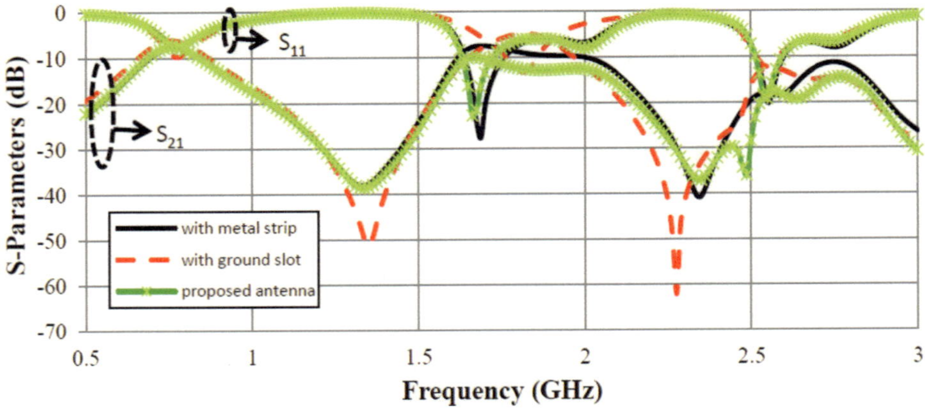

Figure 4. Individual effects of the ground slot and metal strip on *S*-parameter.

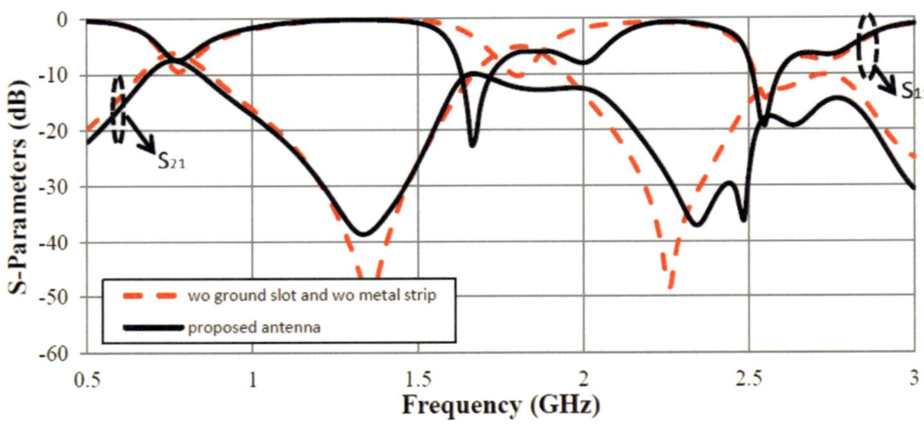

Figure 5. *S*-parameters of the proposed antenna without any isolation techniques and with both the techniques.

3.3. Surface current distribution

Figure 8 shows surface current distributions are shown at 775, 1660, 1810, and 2545 MHz when antenna 1 is excited and antenna 2 is matched terminated. These figures validate the role of slot structure and the metal strip as it is clearly observed that most of the current is present nearby the excited antenna and is trapped in and around the slot structure, thus preventing the flow of current into the second antenna. In this way, the two antennas are less coupled to each other which are the basic requirement of MIMO antenna array.

3.4. 3D far field radiation patterns

The CST MWS is used to plot the 3D far field radiation patterns. The 3D far-field radiation patterns are shown in **Figure 9**. In the case of MIMO antenna system, only one port is excited while keeping other port matched terminated with the 50 Ω load. The radiation patterns

http://dx.doi.org/10.5772/intechopen.75002

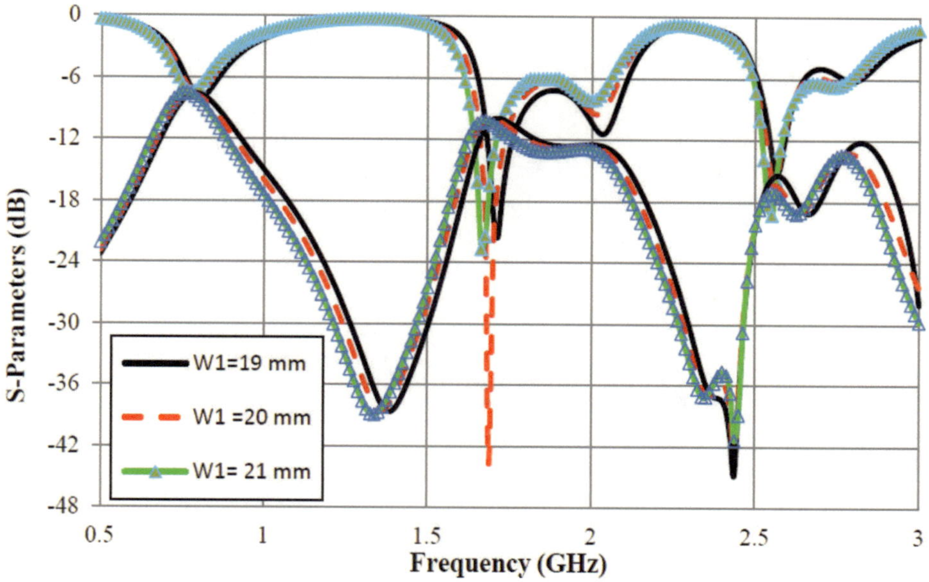

Figure 6. Effect of length 'W_1' on the *S*-parameters.

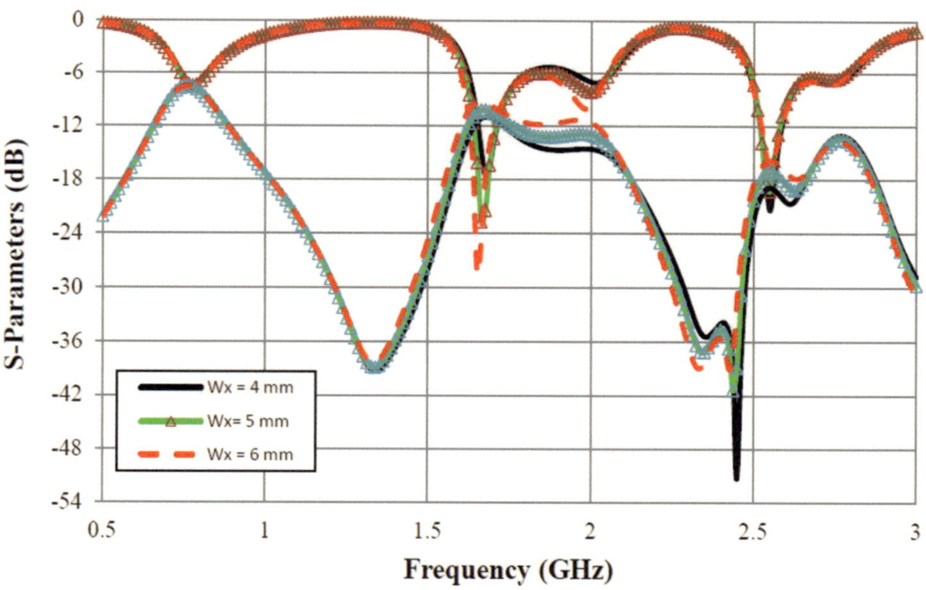

Figure 7. Effect of length 'W_x' on the *S*-parameters.

of Antenna 1 and Antenna 2 are almost mirror images of each other over all the operating frequency bands. That means they are covering the complementary space regions and indicating that the proposed MIMO antenna has good pattern diversity characteristics.

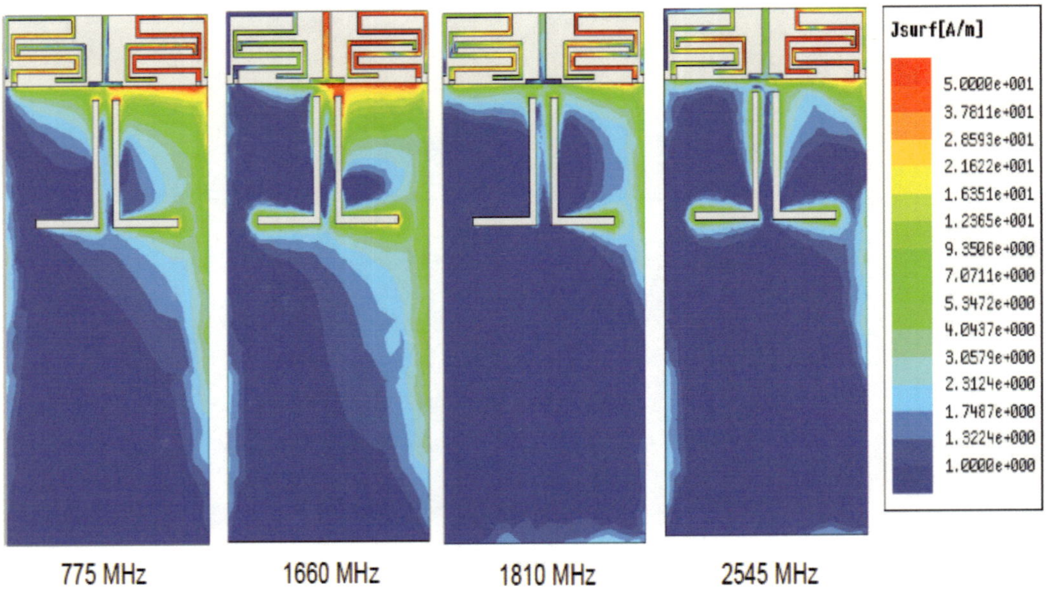

Figure 8. Surface current distributions when the Antenna1 is excited and antenna 2 is matched.

3.5. Diversity characteristics of the proposed antenna

The diversity performance of the proposed MIMO antenna is evaluated by the MEG, correlation coefficient, and diversity gain.

3.5.1. Mean effective gain (MEG)

The MEG values determined MIMO antenna system and given in **Table 2**. The values for MEG1 and MEG2 are almost identical (less than 3 dB difference) and the ratio of MEG1 with MEG2 is close to 1 which satisfies the equality criterion for the two antennas. **Figure 10** shows the computed MEG for Antenna 1 when assuming $mv = mH = 0^\circ$ and $\sigma v = \sigma H = 20^\circ$. It is observed that the computed MEG decreases with increasing the frequency.

3.5.2. Envelope correlation coefficient (ECC)

To evaluate the performance of the proposed MIMO antenna, key performance parameter is ECC. **Figure 11** shows the simulated ECC for the proposed MIMO antenna. The ECC is obtained well below 0.25 for all the operation bands which are practically acceptable.

3.5.3. Diversity gain (DG)

The effectiveness of diversity is given in terms of diversity gain. Diversity gain is calculated using equation (1):

$$DG = \left[\frac{\gamma_c}{\Gamma_c} - \frac{\gamma_1}{\Gamma_1}\right]_{p(\gamma_c < \gamma_s / \Gamma)} \tag{1}$$

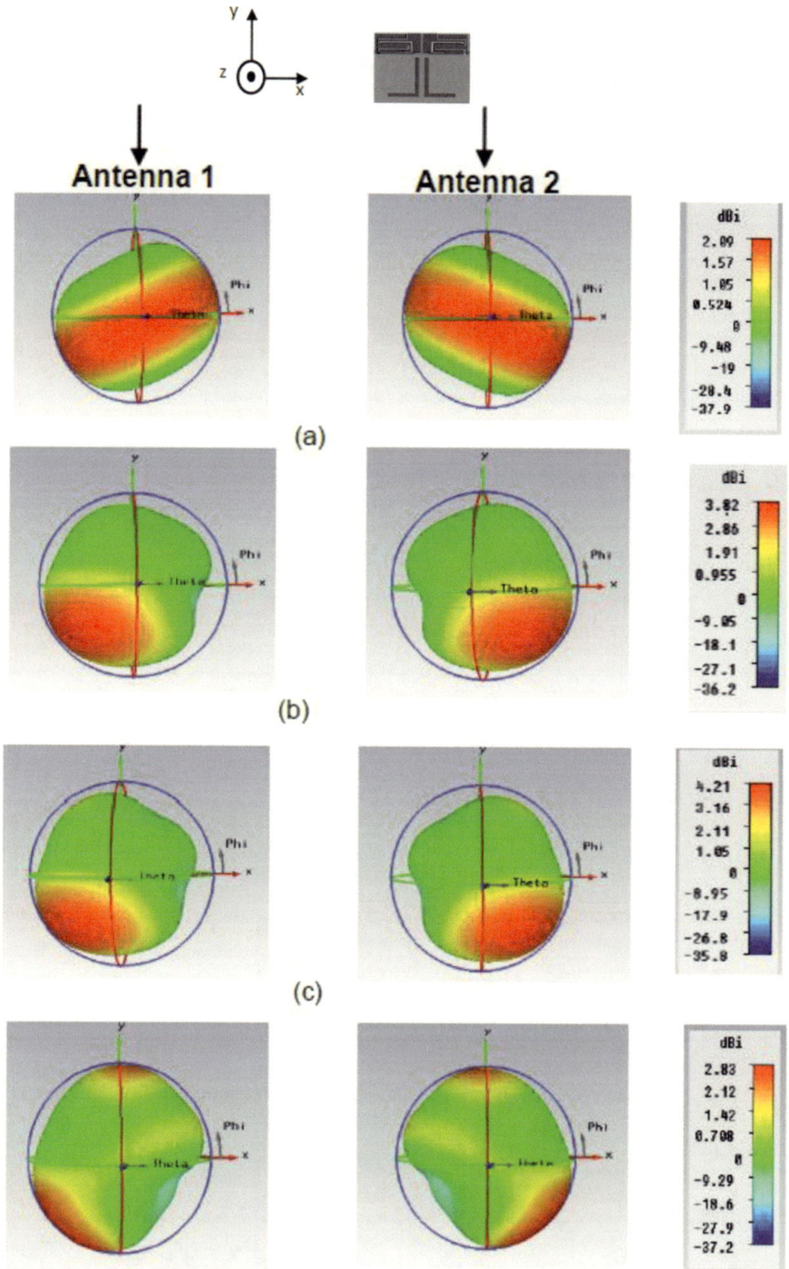

Figure 9. 3D far field radiation patterns at different frequencies (a) 775 MHz, (b) 1660 MHz, (c) 1810 MHz, and (d) 2545 MHz.

where, γ_c is the instantaneous SNR of the diversity combined signal, Γ_c is the mean SNR of the combined signal, γ_1 is the highest SNR of the diversity branch signals, Γ_1 is the mean value of γ_1, and γ_s/Γ is a threshold or reference level.

Mean effective gain	Frequency (GHz)		
	0.77	1.66	2.54
MEG1	−4.3533	−4.8742	−6.0447
MEG2	−4.3625	−4.8624	−6.0210
MEG1/MEG2	0.9978	1.0024	1.0039

Table 2. MEG at different frequencies.

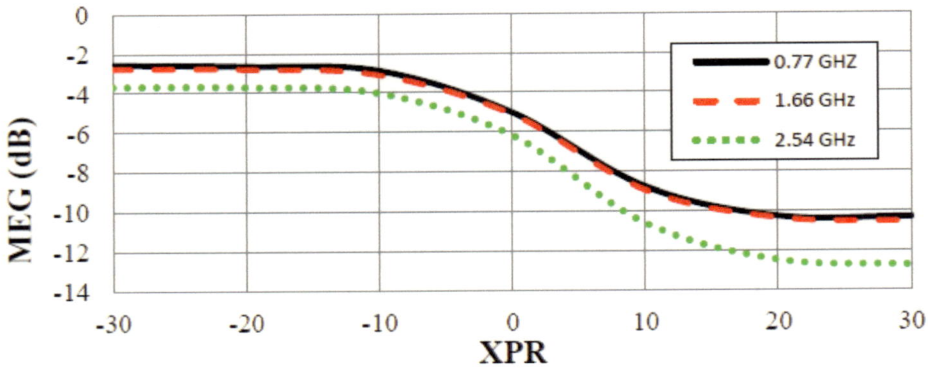

Figure 10. Variation of MEG of antenna 1 with XPR computed.

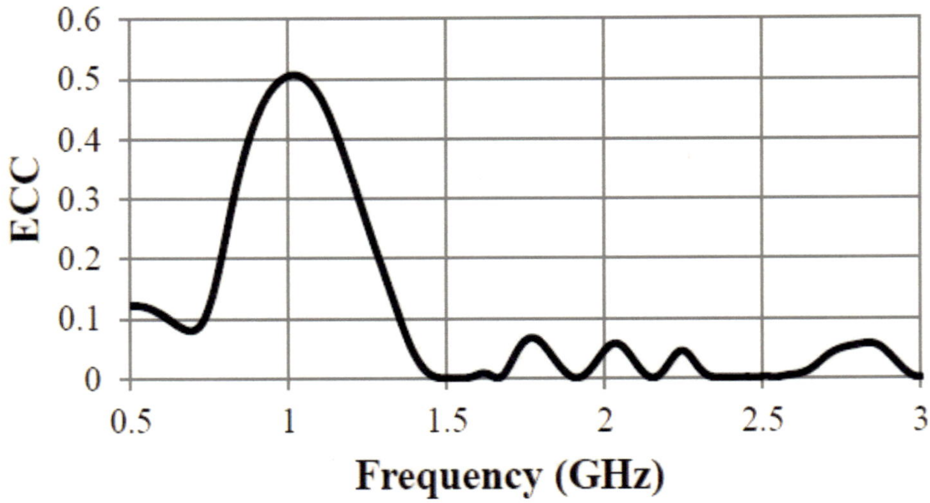

Figure 11. Variation of ECC with frequency.

4. User proximity analysis

4.1. Simulations set-up

The effect of mobile phone configuration (all the major metallic components) is studied for the proposed antenna by keeping the mobile phone antenna at top of the mobile circuit board in talk mode (SAM head and hand). Further, three commonly user style is considered to analyze the user's proximity. **Figure 12(a)** shows talk mode which includes SAM head and PDA hand. Further, to study the data mode (PDA hand) and read mode (dual hand) in addition to the talk mode, the simulation set-up is created in computer simulation technology microwave studio (CST MWS) [14]. **Figure 12(a)** shows two layers head tissue model (fluid and cells) and antenna along with mobile phone configuration (LCD, battery, buttons, speaker, camera, microphones, connectors, and housing) in Talk mode. **Figure 12(b)** shows the hand tissue model and antenna locations for the Data mode. The hand model and holding rules are exactly the same as in the Talk mode, the only difference is that there is no human head model in Data mode. **Figure 12(c)** shows read mode. The user's body *"SAM head and PDA hand (Talk mode)"; "PDA hand (Data mode)" + and position of the mobile phone (antenna with the mobile environment) are in accordance with the cellular telecommunication industry association (CTIA) [15]. Generally, there are three commonly used ways in which users' use their mobile phone i.e. Talk mode, Data mode, and Read mode. In the simulations, human head consists of two layers namely, fluid and cells whereas fluid is confined within the cells and hand model consists of only one layer. The dielectric properties of the human tissue are used in this study can be found in [15]. However, the placement of multi-antenna systems over mobile circuit board is symmetrical with respect to the other mobile circuitry. Hence, any hand of the user (left or right will not cause any difference. In the simulations, we have

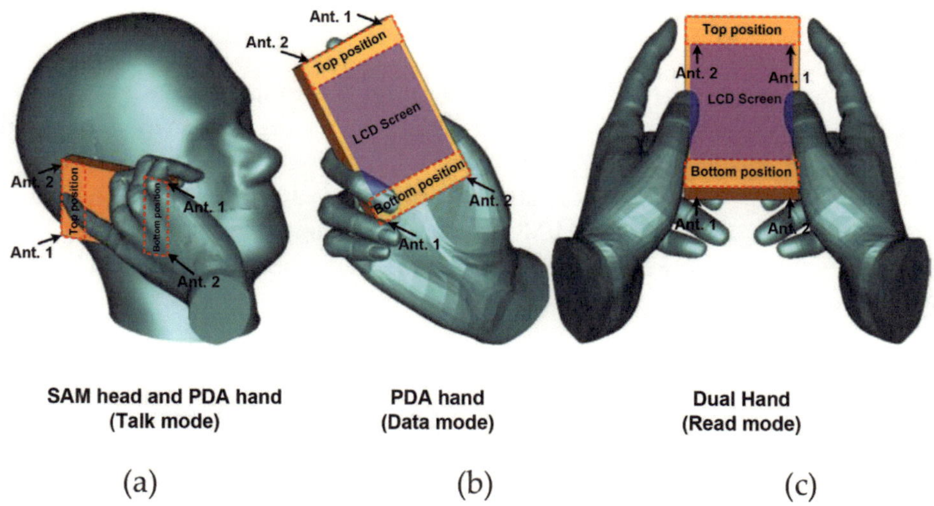

Figure 12. User proximity (a) SAM head and PDA hand, (b) PDA hand, and (c) dual hand.

considered right hand to hold the mobile phone (as most people do). Further, the position of the antenna over mobile circuit board is considered at top and bottom for each case of user proximity. The antenna placed near to the human ear is considered as top position while near to the human mouth is considered as a bottom position of the antenna.

4.2. Channel capacity loss (CCL)

The next important parameters channel capacity loss (CCL) employed to characterize equality of a multi-antenna array. Thus, the CCL is also investigated in free space and user proximity for top and bottom position antenna array. It is computed using *S*-parameter [16] and formula is given as;

$$C_{loss} = -\log_2 \det(\psi_R) \tag{2}$$

where, ψ_R is the receiving antenna correlation matrix. The matrix elements ϱij stands the correlation. The expression shows MIMO systems performance and Closs affect by the reflections at the antenna ports.

$$\psi_R = \begin{pmatrix} \rho_{11} & \rho_{12} \\ \rho_{21} & \rho_{22} \end{pmatrix} \tag{3}$$

here,

$$\rho_{ii} = 1 - |S_{ii}|^2 - |S_{ij}|^2 \tag{4}$$

$$\rho_{ij} = -(S^* ii^* S\, ij + S^* ji^* S\, ij) \quad \text{for } i, j = 1 \text{ or } 2$$

The calculated values of CCL for the multi-antenna array in free space and user proximity are given in **Table 3**. In the free space, the measured CCL is in close agreement with simulated one. Moreover, calculated CCL in user proximity provides high value for the bottom-placed antenna in comparison to the top placed antenna array this is due to high correlation between multi-antenna arrays. For the good MIMO antenna performance, CCL should be less than 0.4 bits/s/Hz. From the **Table 3**, it is depicted that the values are well below 0.4 bits/s/Hz in free space as well as in user proximity.

4.3. Specific absorption rate (SAR) analysis

The effect of radiation from the antenna in human tissues can be evaluated by specific absorption rate (SAR) [15]. The Cellular Telecommunication Industry Association (CTIA) standard is used to calculate the SAR of multi-antenna systems and simulation setup is shown in **Figure 13**. The American standard federal communication commission (FCC) postulate 1.6 W/kg average 1 g tissues, while the European standard postulate 2 W/kg average over 10 g tissues. The stimulating power for SAR calculation is 24 dBm at a lower frequency (0.777 GHz) and 21 dBm for higher frequency (1.9, 2.1, and 2.5 GHz). The calculated values of SAR are given in **Table 4**. As

Frequency (GHz)/Users condition			Antenna at top	Antenna at bottom
0.777	Free space	Simulated	0.37	0.29
		Measured	0.35	0.35
	Talk mode		0.38	0.28
	Data mode		0.3	0.25
	Read mode		0.28	0.2
1.9	Free space	Simulated	0.27	0.21
		Measured	0.21	0.25
	Talk mode		0.24	0.29
	Data mode		0.2	0.19
	Read mode		0.28	0.19
2.1	Free space	Simulated	0.29	0.21
		Measured	0.21	0.29
	Talk mode		0.14	0.13
	Data mode		0.12	0.12
	Read mode		0.14	0.12
2.5	Free space	Simulated	0.2	0.21
		Measured	0.24	0.21
	Talk mode		0.19	0.15
	Data mode		0.17	0.17
	Read mode		0.14	0.18

Table 3. Variation of CCL in free space and user proximity.

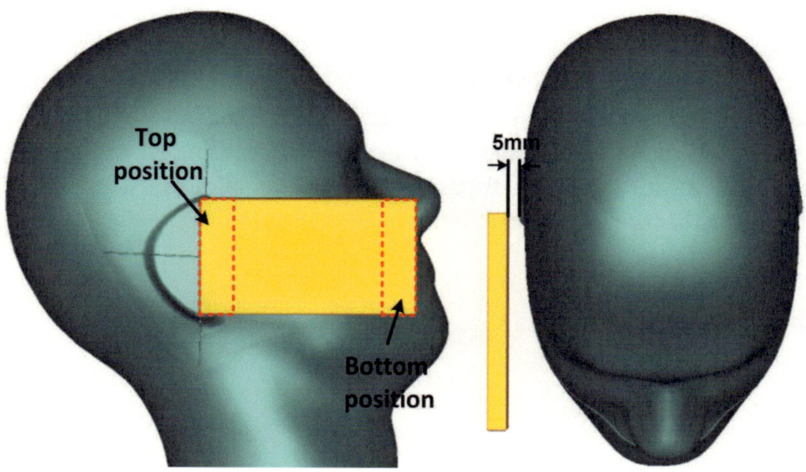

Figure 13. SAR setup according to CTIA.

Antenna	Freq.	0.777 GHz	1.9 GHz	2.1 GHz	2.5 GHz
		Top position			
Ant. 1 (W/kg)	FCC	0.6	0.7	0.78	0.49
	European	0.29	0.31	0.43	0.21
Ant. 2 (W/kg)	FCC	0.7	1.2	0.95	0.68
	European	0.42	0.37	0.64	0.29
		Bottom position			
Ant. 1 (W/kg)	FCC	0.38	0.39	0.24	0.33
	European	0.38	0.29	0.28	0.15
Ant. 2 (W/kg)	FCC	0.42	0.38	0.37	0.24
	European	0.3	0.29	0.27	0.21

Table 4. SAR values for the head phantom.

per the simulation setup, the distance between head phantom and the bottom-placed antenna is more, result in lower SAR while top located antenna provides larger SAR values. It is interestingly noted that lower SAR values are achieved for both standards because of the plastic box cover the mobile phone antenna. It can also be observed that SAR values of Ant. 1 and Ant. 2 is slightly different for top and bottom placed elements due to non-planar phantom. The calculated values of SAR follow the defined standard.

5. Conclusion

In this chapter, a quad-band monopole MIMO antenna covering LTE13/14, GSM1800, PCS1900, and LTE2600 is presented. The proposed antenna consists of an antenna and parasitic plate which resonates at 762, 1787, and 2550 MHz with good return loss. By introducing the vertical plate shifting of lower frequency from 937 to 762 MHz is observed. Enhancement of bandwidth and isolation is observed by cutting slot on the ground and by placing the metal strip in between the antennas. With these features, as well as compact and simple configuration, the proposed MIMO antenna is appropriate for the mobile handsets. The study of user proximity confirms that the proposed antenna suitable for mobile handsets.

Author details

Hari Shankar Singh

Address all correspondence to: harishankar1990@gmail.com

Department of Electronics and Communication Engineering, Thapar Institute of Engineering and Technology, Patiala, Punjab, India

References

[1] Chiau CC. Study of the diversity antenna array for the MIMO wireless communication systems. [Ph. D. Thesis] UK: University of London; 2006

[2] Paulraj A, Gore D, Nabar R, Bolcskei H. An overview of MIMO communications–a key to gigabit wireless. Proceedings of the IEEE. 2004;**92**:198-218. DOI: 10.1109/JPROC.2003.821915

[3] Farhadi H, Wang C, Skoglund M. Distributed transceiver design and power control for wireless MIMO interference networks. IEEE Transactions on Wireless Communications. 2014;**14**:1199-1212. DOI: 10.1109/TWC.2014.2365202

[4] Ogawa K, Uwano T. A diversity antenna for very small 800-MHz band portable telephones. IEEE Transactions on Antennas and Propagation. 1994;**42**:1342-1345. DOI: 10.1109/8.318664

[5] Jensen MA, Samii YR. Performance analysis of antennas for hand-held transceivers using FDTD. IEEE Transactions on Antennas and Propagation. 1994;**42**:1106-1113. DOI: 10.1109/8.310002

[6] Singh HS, Meruva B, Pandey GK, Bharti PK, Meshram MK. Low mutual coupling between MIMO antennas by using two folded shorting strips. Progress in Electromagnetics Research B. 2013;**205-221**(2013):53. DOI: 10.2528/PIERB13052305

[7] Vaughan RG, Andersen JB. Antenna diversity in mobile communications. IEEE Transactions on Vehicular Technology. 2013;**VT-36**:149-172. DOI: 10.1109/T-VT.1987.24115

[8] Sesia S, Toufik I, Baker M. LTE-The UMTS Long Term Evolution: From Theory to Practice. Chichester, U.K.: Wiley; 2009. DOI: 10.1002/9780470742891

[9] Wong K, Kang T, Tu M. Internal mobile phone antenna array for LTE/WWAN and LTE MIMO operations. Microwave and Optical Technology Letters. 2011;**53**:156-157. DOI: 10.1002/mop.26038

[10] Sharawi MS, Faouri YS, Iqbal SS. Design and fabrication of a dual electrically small MIMO antenna system for 4G terminals. In: Proceedings of the 6th German Microwave Conference; 14-16 March 2011. Darmstadt, Germany: IEEE; 2011. pp. 1-4

[11] Zhang S, Zhao K, Ying Z, He S. Diagonal antenna-chassis mode and its application for wideband LTE MIMO antennas in mobile handsets. In: Proceeding of International Workshop on Antenna Technology (iWAT); 4-6 March 2013. Sweden: IEEE; 2013. pp. 1-4. DOI: 10.1109/IWAT.2013.6518376

[12] Shen SD, Guo T, Kuang F, Zhang X, Wu K. A novel wideband printed diversity antenna for mobile handsets. In: Proceeding IEEE 75th Vehicular Technology Conference (VTC Spring); 6-9 May 2012. Yokohama: IEEE; 2012. pp. 1-5. DOI: 10.1109/VETECS.2012.6240173

[13] Singh HS, Bharti P, Pandey GK, Meshram MK. A compact tri-band MIMO/diversity antenna for mobile handsets. In: Proceeding IEEE CONECCT; 17-19 January 2013. Bangalore, India: IEEE; 2013. pp. 1-6. DOI: 10.1109/CONECCT.2013.6469306

[14] Computer Simulation Technology Microwave Studio (CST MWS), [Online] available: http://www.cst.com

[15] "Test plan for mobile station over the air performance," CTIA revision 3.1, January 2011

[16] Choukiker YK, Sharma SK, Behera SK. Hybrid fractal shape planar monopole antenna covering multiband wireless communications with MIMO implementation for handheld mobile devices. IEEE Transactions on Antennas and Propagation. 2014;(3):1483-1488. DOI: 10.1109/TAP.2013.2295213

Chapter 3

Wireless Body Area Networking: Joint Physical-Networking Layer Simulation and Modeling

Mojtaba Fallahpour

Additional information is available at the end of the chapter

http://dx.doi.org/10.5772/intechopen.79251

Abstract

An electronic device equipped with sensors and antennas is the main part of the wireless body area networking (WBAN). Such a device is placed near human body and it usually works in a populated environment with many surrounding objects (e.g., building walls). The human body and the objects can change the radiation characteristics of the antenna and impact the performance of the wireless communication system. The wireless communication system's performance is also affected by the networking layers established on top of the physical layer. Therefore, any designing method for WBAN application should be pervasive, offering a joint physical-networking layer simulation and modeling strategy. To this end, in this chapter, a comprehensive simulation and modeling method is presented. First, antenna design limitations and challenges for wireless body area networking are studied with emphasis on evaluating the antenna's performance near the human body. Then, the antenna miniaturization techniques to reduce the antennas' dimension are reviewed. Later, a system level analysis and modeling are used to study short-range communication between the wearable antennas with remote nodes using IEEE 802.11g wireless networking protocol.

Keywords: wearable antenna, miniaturization, modeling, WBAN

1. Introduction

The growing interest in using connected sensors for health-care related medical diagnoses and screening demands a proper communication backbone to establish wireless body area networking (WBAN). Miniaturized electronic devices touching or placed very close to the human body are essential parts of the WBAN. These devices are equipped with sensors and can collect data about different health-related parameters (e.g., blood sugar) in real-time [1–4]. The collected data are processed by the device itself or transmitted to another device (node) or cloud for further processing and decision-making. In order to have communication between the devices, several networking layers should be established and optimized. The physical layer is responsible for delivering data (digital bits) from sender to the destination. This backbone layer includes hardware (i.e., transmitter, receiver and antenna) and propagation medium (or channel). Other layers are built over this layer and create the connectivity and ability to communicate. The antenna is vital for wireless communication. The antenna's performance is dictated by several factors including its electrical length (physical length normalized to the operating wavelength) and the surrounding medium. For the antennas working in the microwave regime, the wavelength is measured in the centimeter scale, and so the minimum antenna dimension is usually limited to a few centimeters. On the other hand, available integrated circuit design technologies allow the whole electronics section (including sensors and processing units) to be made as small as a few millimeters. This clearly shows that the antenna is currently a bottleneck for developing small size wireless devices for WBAN.

In this chapter, first, antenna design limitations and challenges for wireless body area networking are studied with emphasis on evaluating the antenna's performance near the human body. Several antenna miniaturization techniques are reviewed, which can be used to reduce the antennas' dimension.

Later, a system-level analysis and modeling are invoked to study short-range communication between the wearable antennas with remote nodes using IEEE 802.11 g wireless networking protocol.

2. Wearable antennas

Designing a small size, flexible, body conformal, and biocompatible antenna is critical for WBAN applications. Achieving a reasonable gain (and efficiency) while reducing the antenna's dimensions is challenging [5–8]. Here, design and optimization of a typical patch antenna on a flexible PCB and its performance near the human body is studied. Three different human body models are considered: a planar slab with homogenous material (Model 1), multilayered (Model 2) and the whole-body model (Model 3).

2.1. Modeling the human body

The human body is made of different materials with different electrical (e.g., dielectric constant (permittivity) and conductivity), physical (e.g., thickness) and mechanical (e.g., compressibility, mass density) properties. Most of the electronic devices are relatively small and therefore the area directly in contact or near the device is the most influential part. Hence, the simplest model for a human body to be used for studying the electromagnetic wave interaction can be a homogenous dielectric slab. The dielectric constant for the slab is calculated by performing an averaging on the dielectric properties of the different parts (i.e., skin, fat, muscle, etc.). This model is shown in **Figure 1(a)** and is called Model 1.

Considering the simplicity of Model 1, it may not completely capture and model the wave propagation inside a human body. Hence, a four-layer model is also included in this study (**Figure 1(b)**). The first (exterior) layer is skin, the second layer is fat, and the third layer is tissue. Depending on which part of the body is investigated, more layers including organs (e.g., heart or kidney) or bone can be added to the model. Thickness of layers is represented as $t_{layer\ name}$. This model is referred to as Model 2.

Modeling the whole body with all the details and features is computationally costly, but sometimes is needed (e.g., to evaluate the interaction of multiple devices installed on different parts of the body). The human body's electrical properties are usually frequency dependent and can significantly change at the microwave/millimeter wave regimes. Hence, characterizing and predicting these behaviors are vital for modeling purposes. Fortunately, in the recent years, there has been a great progress in this regard, and the electrical properties of different organs and tissues are included in commercial simulation tools such as ANSYS HFSS [9]. ANSYS's available 3D human body models (**Figure 2(a)**) include internal organs (e.g., the lung). For these simulations, the wearable antenna is placed outside the body, and to avoid the computational complexity during the simulations, the model with homogenous average material is used and referred to as Model 3 (**Figure 2(b)**).

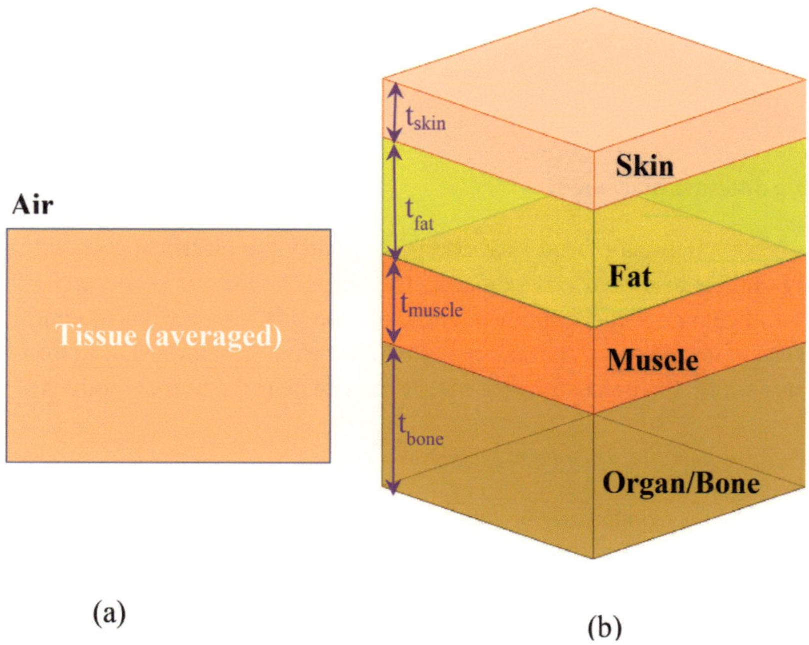

Figure 1. Flat models for human body: (a) model 1: homogenous dielectric slab and (b) model 2: multilayered structure.

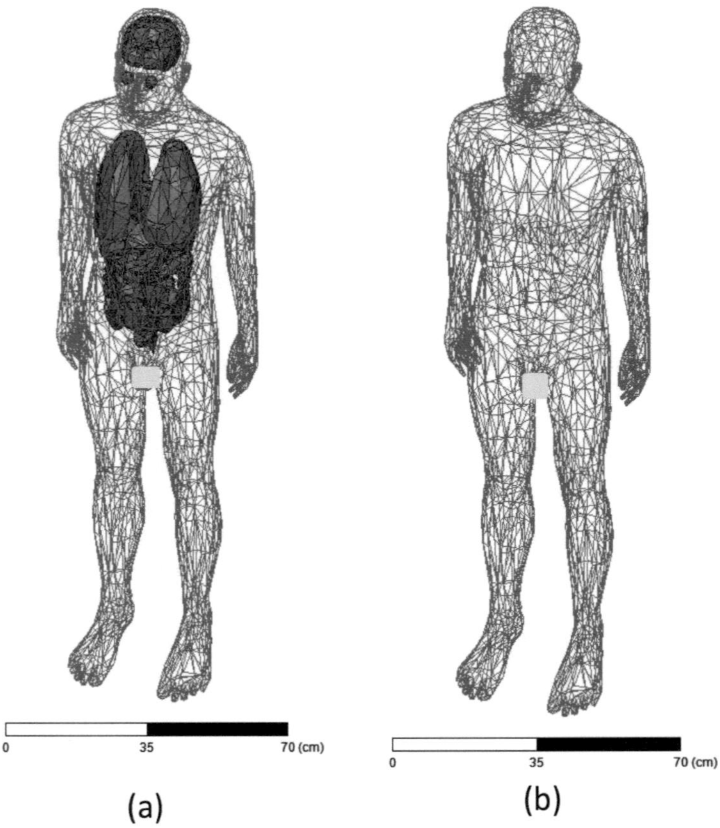

Figure 2. Human body models included in ASNSY HFSS (version R18.2). (a) Complete model with internal organs and (b) model 3: homogenous model.

2.2. Wearable antenna placement

For the wearable antennas placed near the body (skin), the electrical contrast between the human body and air results in wave reflections. Hence, the human body can load the radiating antenna and change its performance. The radiation pattern, gain, and radiation efficiency are some of the main radiation characteristics which define the antenna's performance. In the following case study, the patch antenna's performance near the human body is studied.

2.2.1. Flexible patch antenna: design and evaluation

The patch antenna is popular among antenna engineers because of its ease of fabrication and integration with planar geometries. The recent development of flexible printed circuits (FPCs) makes it possible to create wearable conformal patch antennas [10]. In this section, design and evaluation of a patch antenna operating at 2.4 GHz and implemented on a FPC will be studied. The geometry of the antenna is shown in **Figure 3**. Double sided FPC polyamide film material is selected for the antenna implementation. The substrate thickness (h) is 1 mm and its dielectric constant and dielectric loss tangent are $\varepsilon_r = 4.3$ and $\tan\delta = 0.004$, respectively.

http://dx.doi.org/10.5772/intechopen.79251

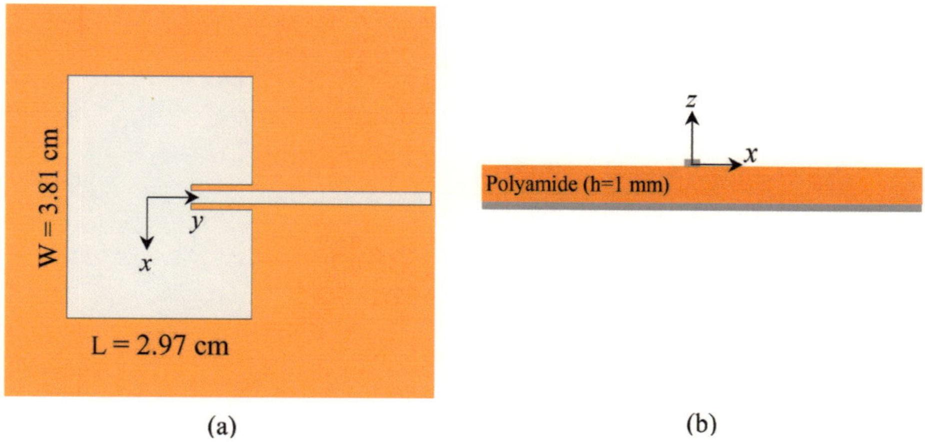

Figure 3. Designed patch antenna on FPC polyamide film material: (a) front view and (b) side view.

The patch antenna with edge feeding was initially designed to operate in free-space. To achieve the desired matching at 2.4 GHz, ANSYS HFSS was used to model, simulate, tune and optimize the dimensions and feed line location and configuration (listed in **Figure 3**). The antenna's input impedance matching to 50 Ω reference impedance, presented as the reflection coefficient (S_{11}), is plotted in **Figure 4**, which shows a good impedance matching at 2.4 GHz. The antenna's radiation gain pattern (3D) is shown in **Figure 5(a)**. The peak realized

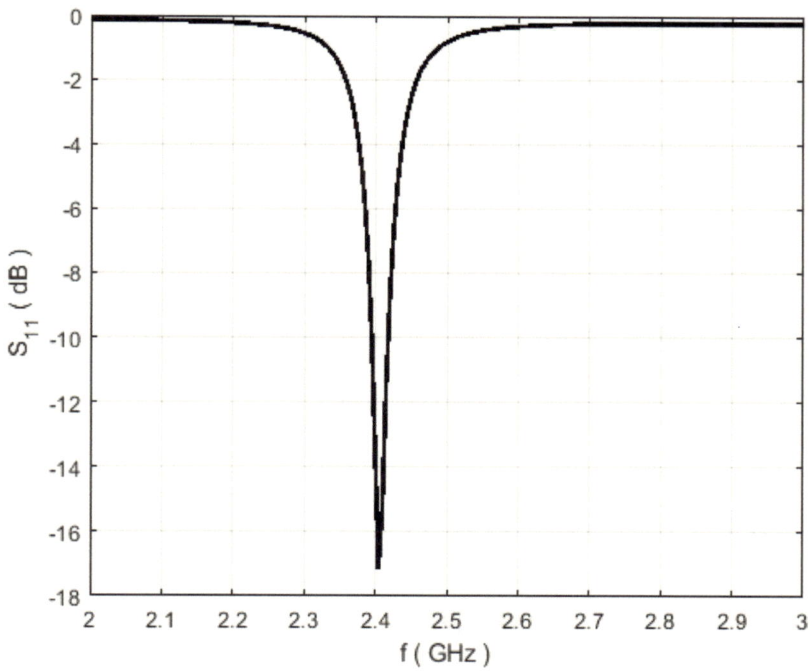

Figure 4. Calculated return loss for the flexible patch antenna from HFSS simulation.

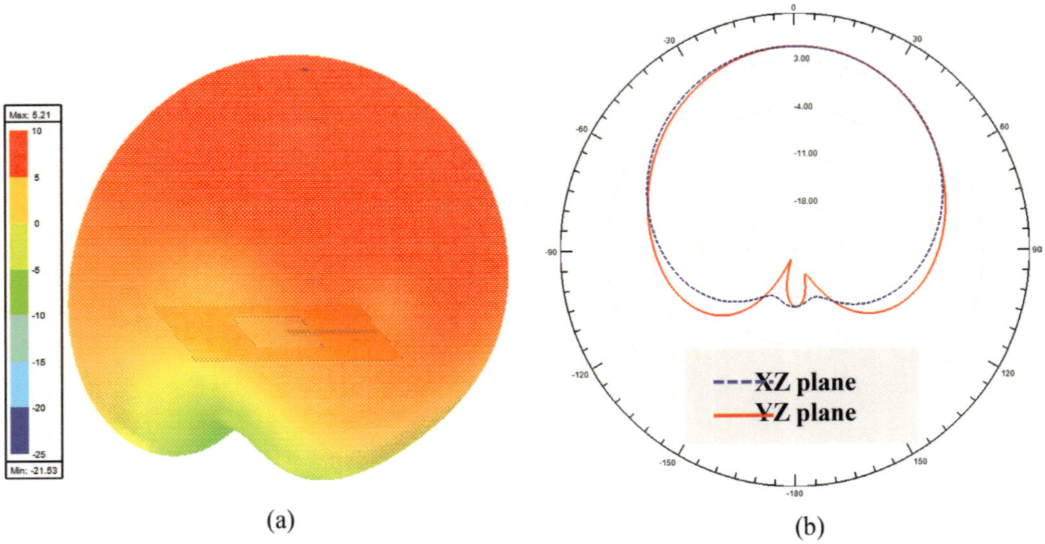

Figure 5. Patch antenna's radiation gain pattern: (a) 3D view and (b) polar plot at XZ and YZ planes (scale: dB).

gain value (including matching loss) is 3.24 dB and the radiation efficiency is 71%. Moreover, the radiation pattern at two orthogonal planes XZ and YZ is extracted from the 3D plot and shown in **Figure 5(b)**. The plots show that the antenna has a directional beam pointing to the forward direction. Therefore, the front to back ration (F/B) for the radiation pattern is relatively high (21 dB). The antenna's characteristics are summarized in **Table 1**.

In the second step, the antenna was placed near the human body (stand-off distance of 4 mm), where Model 1 was used to represent the human body (ε_r = 28.5, σ = 3 S/m). The overall radiation performance is slightly impacted and changed (see **Table 1**). In fact, the human body acted as a large lossy reflector, and reflected the energy, resulting in a more directional beam.

Later, the antenna was placed on a four-layer model (Model 2) with stand-off distance of 4 mm and the performance was investigated. The layer properties were set as dry skin (ε_r = 36, t_{skin} = 0.1 cm), fat (ε_r = 5.27, t_{fat} = 0.5), muscle (ε_r = 52.6, t_{muscle} = 4 cm) and bone (ε_r = 18.4, t_{bone} = half-space extension). The antenna's radiation performance is summarized in **Table 1**. Like the previous case, there are some slight changes.

Configuration	f (GHz)	Realized gain (dB)	Radiation efficiency (%)	F/B ratio (dB)
Antenna in free-space	2.4	3.24	71	21
Antenna near Model 1	2.4	4.82	65	19
Antenna near Model 2	2.4	4.76	61	27
Antenna near Model 3	2.4	4.22	61	26

Table 1. Comparing the designed patch antenna's performance for different scenarios.

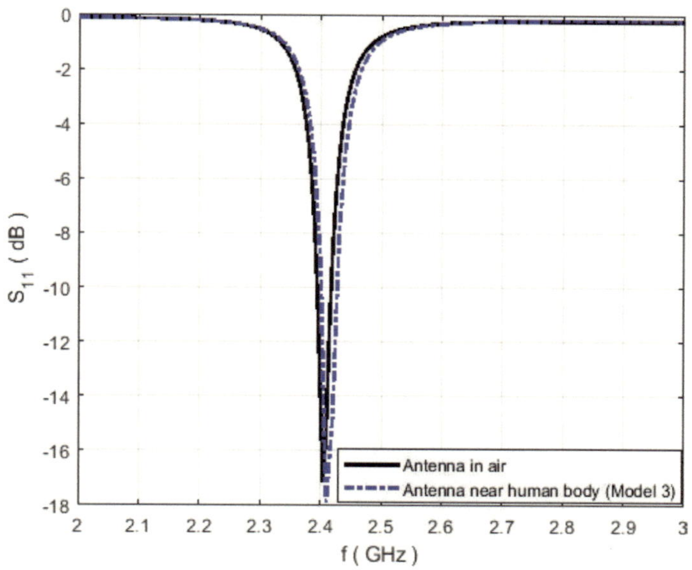

Figure 6. Simulated return loss for the flexible patch antenna placed on the left arm of the human body model (model 3) compared with the results for the antenna placed in air.

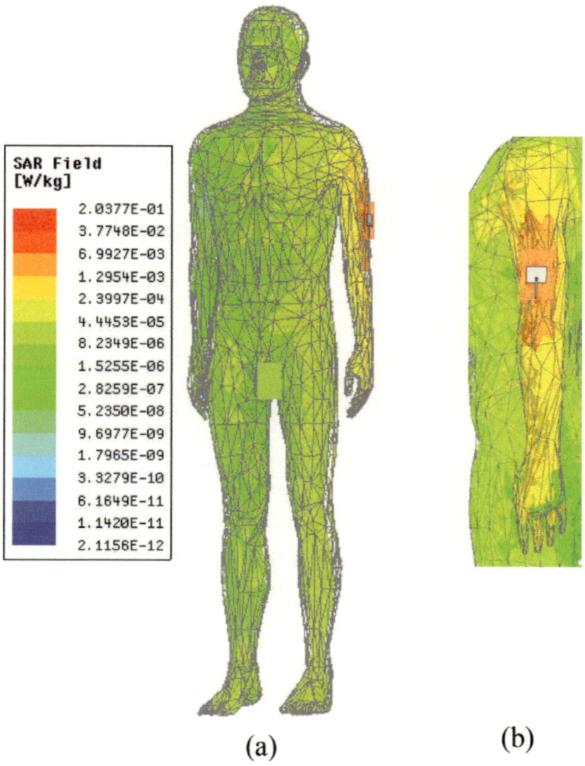

Figure 7. HFSS simulated average SAR distribution (W/kg) at 2.4 GHz (total absorbed power of 0.9 mW), (a) full-view, (b) selected left hand with the radiating antenna.

Finally, the antenna was placed on the left arm of the human body (Model 3) and its performance was investigated using the HFSS simulation tool and the results are listed in **Table 1**. The resonance frequency is shifted from 2.4 GHz to 2.41 GHz (**Figure 6**), but the overall performance of the antenna at 2.4 GHz is still acceptable.

From a safety point of view, the amount of heat generated by the antenna radiation is usually reported in term of the specific absorption rate (SAR). For the current example, the calculated average SAR is presented in **Figure 7**. There are different safety regulations and limits imposed by different countries. For example, in the United States, "the Federal Communications Commission (FCC) limit for public exposure from cellular telephones is an SAR level of 1.6 watts per kilogram (1.6 W/kg)" [11]. All wireless device manufacturers should obey this regulation. For the current example, for 10 mW available power from source, 8.80 mW was accepted by the patch antenna. From this 8.8 mW, 5.4 mW radiated, and 3.4 mW was dissipated in term of heat by the antenna and human body. The simulation results show that 0.9 mW was absorbed by the body and 2.5 mW was dissipated by the antenna itself.

3. Antenna miniaturization

Size reduction (beside conformality) is one of the main challenges in designing wearable antennas. In this section, some of the antenna miniaturization techniques will be reviewed.

Miniaturization techniques: In general, an antenna's properties and characteristics can be modified by altering its geometry, current density distribution, materials and electrical dimensions [5–7]. The antenna characteristics are usually defined in terms of input impedance matching, radiation pattern, gain, polarization, efficiency, quality (Q)-factor, and band width. In the past several decades, antenna miniaturization methods have been developed that efficiently modify and optimize the shape and the overall geometry of an antenna in order to achieve the desired characteristics while limiting the overall dimensions to be as small as possible. The miniaturization methods can be divided into topology-based and material-based methods. The topology-based techniques mainly focus on finding proper topology (e.g., geometry) for the antenna to improve its characteristics, while the material-based techniques usually achieve the desired characteristics by changing the antenna's materials (e.g., using high dielectric constant substrates). Each category has several members. Some of them are discussed here, but a more complete discussion can be found in [5].

(A) Meander antennas: Meander antennas aim to efficiently fill the available space by bending a long line to create a current distribution with proper phase and amplitude variations (**Figure 8**) [5]. The antenna's resonance frequency can be lowered by adding more bending to a fixed straight line. However, the radiation performance (e.g., peak gain) may decrease as a result of meandering. This is mainly because the arms can carry opposing currents whose radiation cancel each other in the far field region. Moreover, by increasing the length, the ohmic loss may increase. Meander antennas are used in commercial products due to their compactness and low manufacturing cost. As an example, meander antennas are used to design miniaturized ultra-high frequency (UHF) radio frequency identification (RFID) tags [12]. These tags are becoming popular in WBAN applications [13]. Overall, applying the meandering concept to design wearable antennas can help reduce the size of the antenna.

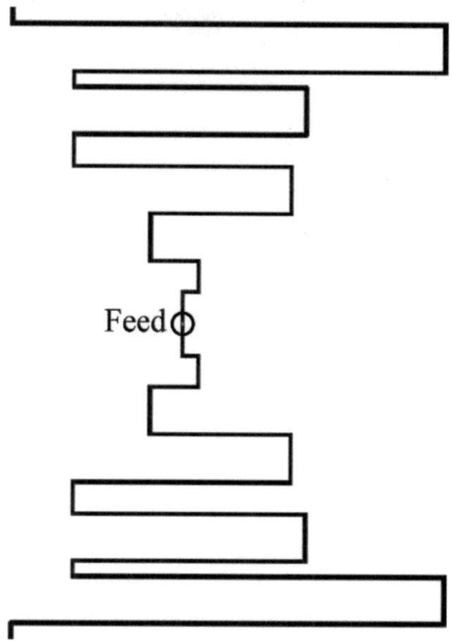

Figure 8. A meander dipole antenna.

(B) Fractal antennas: Fractals are geometrical objects that exhibit a repeating pattern on many different length scales. Very long fractal curves can be fit into a relatively small area. This feature of the fractals, in addition to their self-similarity, attracted antenna engineers and has been used by them to create a new class of antennas, called fractal antennas [5]. The multiband performance and compactness of the fractal antennas make them a good candidate for wearable designs [14]. For example, the Koch fractal geometry can be used to design compact dipole antennas (**Figure 9**).

(C) Reactively loaded antennas: Boundary conditions applied to an antenna can be modified in a way to change its resonance frequency. This can be done by adding a shorting pin or

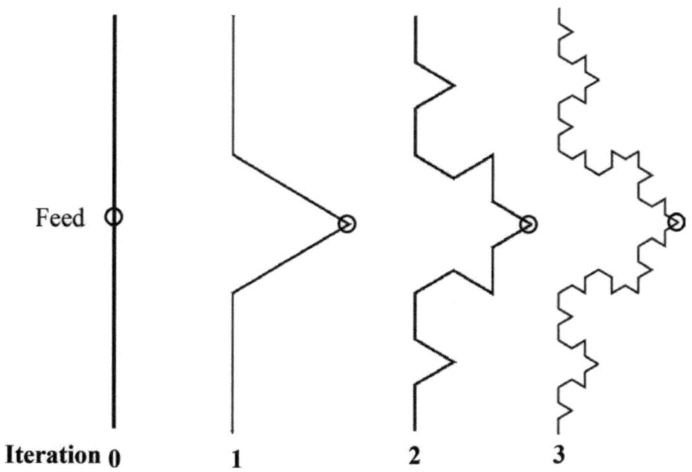

Figure 9. Different iterations of Koch dipole antenna.

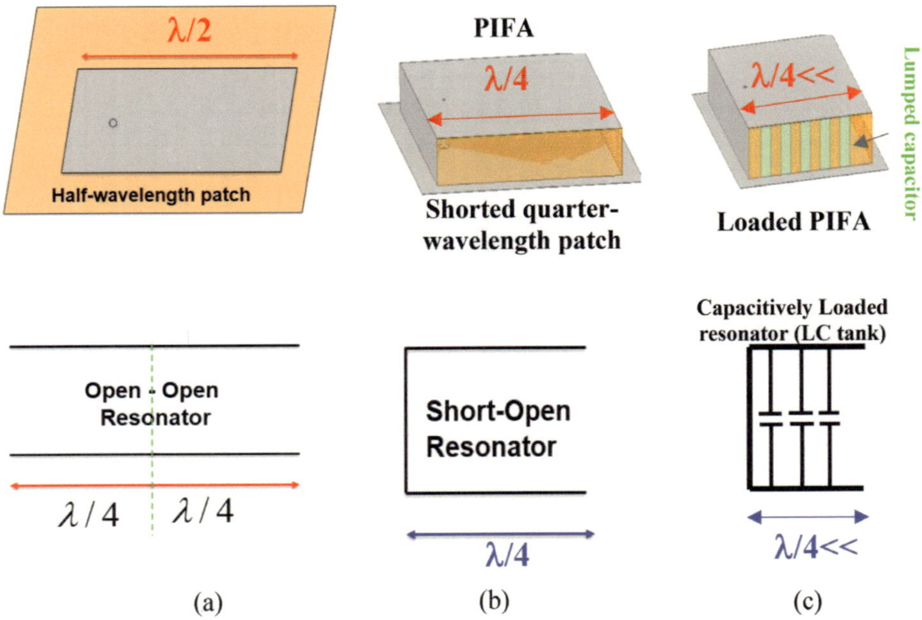

Figure 10. Miniaturing a conventional patch antenna: (a) the patch and its resonator model, (b) shorted quarter-wavelength patch (or PIFA) and its equivalent resonator model and (c) loaded PIFA and its resonator model.

loading the antenna with appropriate lumped or distributed inductors or capacitors. For example, a half-wave patch antenna is an open-open resonator (**Figure 10(a)**). By shorting one of the radiating sides of the patch using a metallic plate or vias, an open-short resonator is created (**Figure 10(b)**). This new resonator can resonate at a lower frequency compared to the open-open resonator. This is the idea behind planar inverted-F antennas (PIFAs). In addition, by loading the nonradiating sides with lumped capacitors, one can create a slow-wave structure and further lower the resonance frequency (**Figure 10(c)**) [5]. This type of antennas can be electrically very small; however, the cost is gain and radiation efficiency degradation.

4. Modeling IEEE 802.11 g wireless network

To establish a successful communication between the wearable device with other wireless devices or the base station (or in general node to node communication), the physical layer provides a backbone, and other layers will be formed on this layer. Having a pervasive simulation tool which can combine different modalities and model different layers simultaneously is invaluable to study the wireless communication between nodes. Fortunately, in recent years, there has been significant progress in commercial simulation tools to realize a bottom to top system level modeling and simulation capability. In this section, ANSYS tools will be used to simulate and study the communication between a wearable antenna and a remote node using the IEEE 802.11 g wireless networking standard. Both nodes are assumed to be inside a building (indoor) where the multiple multipath reflections and attenuation makes the wireless communication more challenging.

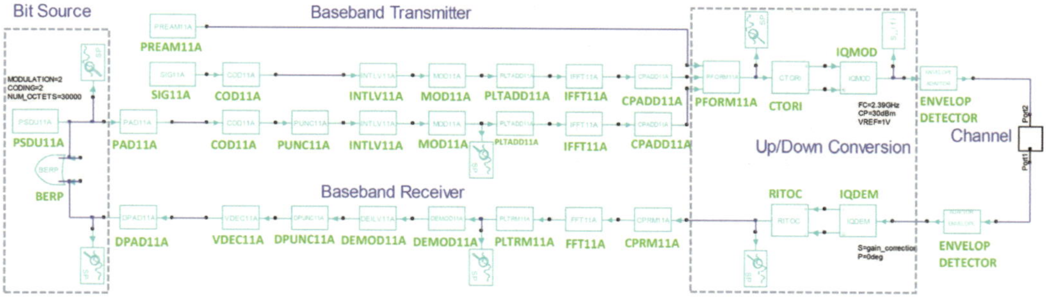

Figure 11. IEEE 802.11 g schematic view inside ANSYS circuit simulator [8].

System-Level Modeling: The entire block diagram for the 802.11 g wireless networking system, available inside the ANSYS Circuit simulator (R18.2), is shown in **Figure 11**. Five different sections can be recognized in this implementation. The source section is responsible for generating the bit stream. The baseband transmitter encodes and modulates the digital bits. The Up/Down conversion section puts the digital signal on a carrier frequency (f_C = 2.4 GHz) in the transmitter side. This section will down-convert the received signal to a baseband signal. The channel represents both transmitter and receiver antennas and the propagation medium between them. In other words, it captures the wave propagation from transmitter to receiver over the wireless communication medium (e.g., building interior).

The channel model can be imported as a scattering matrix [S] from simulation or measurement. For a two-port network (i.e., single transmitter, single receiver), the [S] matrix has four entries (S_{11},S_{12},S_{21},S_{22}), and it describes the device/network behavior when it is exposed to the electromagnetic waves. In general, scattering parameters are used to model linear network behavior at high frequencies, and they include valuable information about the device including impedance matching at the ports, insertion loss and delay between the ports. For indoor applications, the environment includes human body, walls, windows, desk, chair, floor and many other objects (**Figure 12**). Therefore, the environment is electrically large, and the chance of multiple and multipath reflections is high. To model such a large problem, the ANSYS Savant tool was used and the communication between the wearable antenna and the wireless node is studied for two

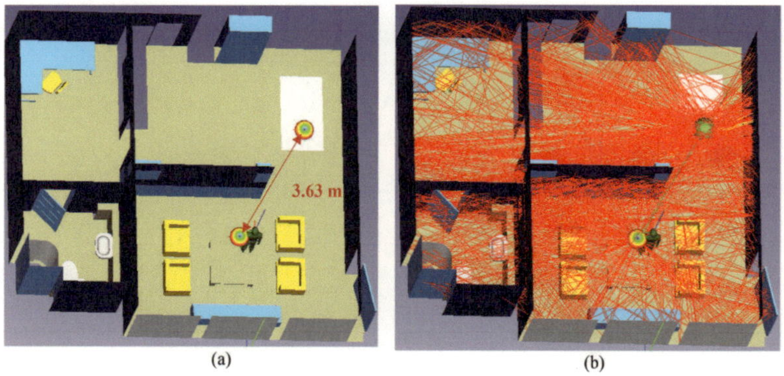

Figure 12. Line of sight indoor communication between wearable device and a remote node modeled in ANSYS Savant: (a) the whole scenario and (b) virtual ray tracing from transmitter to receiver.

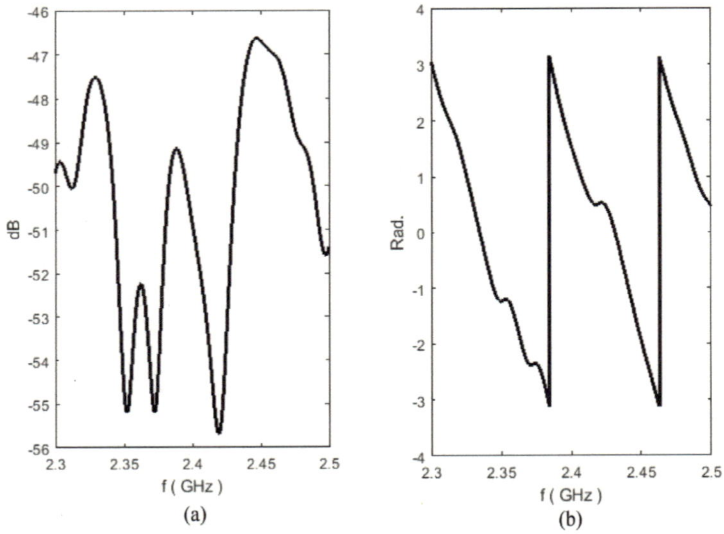

Figure 13. ANSYS Savant's simulation result for coupling between the transmitter and receiver nodes for line of sight indoor communication scenario: (a) magnitude in dB and (b) phase in radians.

configurations. For the antennas, half-wave dipoles operating at 2.4 GHz are used. The wearable antenna is called node 1, and the remote external node is named as node 2.

Case 1: In the first scenario, both nodes are positioned at line of sight distance of 3.63 m (**Figure 12(a)**). The simulation was performed in Savant using the shooting and bouncing rays (SBR) technique. The transmitter node (i.e., the wearable antenna) shoots several rays per wavelength. These rays can directly reach to the receiver or arrive with delay after bouncing from the objects (**Figure 12(b)**). The scattering parameter S_{21} (magnitude and phase) which has information about the channel loss/delay is shown in **Figure 13**. Then, the scattering matrix was imported to the ANSYS Circuit simulator and used to simulate the IEEE 802.11 g wireless networking between the nodes. To have a more realistic scenario, white Gaussian noise (WGN) was generated using an external source block, and it was added to the channel's output using sum operator. The carrier

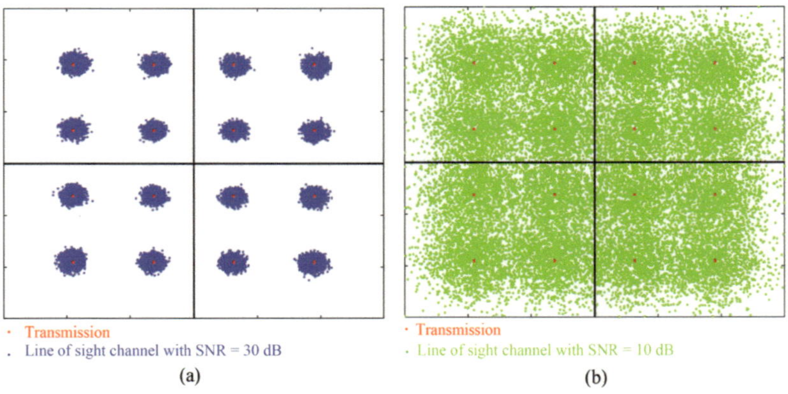

Figure 14. Simulation result for QAM-16 constellation plot at the receiver node for Case 1 (line of sight scenario): (a) SNR = 30 dB and (b) SNR = 10 dB.

http://dx.doi.org/10.5772/intechopen.79251

signal's power was set to 1 W (30 dBm) and the QAM-16 constellation plot for two different signal-to-noise ratio (SNR) values of 30 and 10 dB are shown in **Figure 14(a)** and **(b)**, respectively. By reducing the SNR to 10 dB, the constellation plot is no longer acceptable.

Case 2: In the second scenario, the nodes are positioned in two rooms separated by walls (nonline of sight scenario) at distance of 7.2 m (**Figure 15(a)**). The rays could only make their way from transmitter to receiver through walls and/or multiple bouncing (**Figure 15(b)**). From the calculated S_{21} in **Figure 16**, it can be seen that the multipath and multiple reflections created an interference pattern and negatively impacted the received signal's strength at the desired frequency range. This shows itself in the constellation plot (**Figure 17**) where the received signals are not categorized properly for SNR as high as 90 dB.

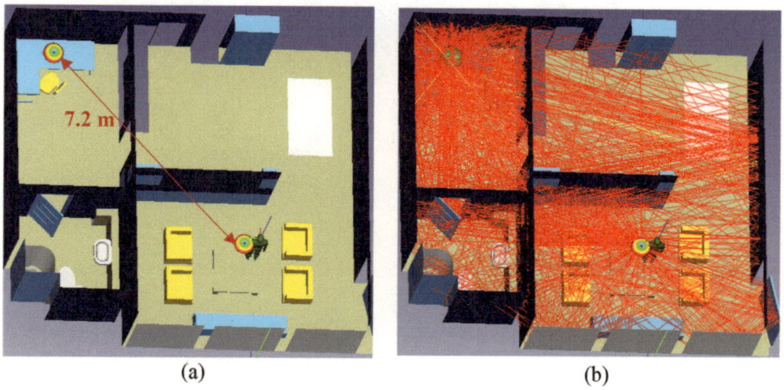

Figure 15. Nonline of sight indoor communication between wearable device and a remote node modeled in ANSYS Savant: (a) the whole scenario and (b) virtual ray tracing from transmitter to receiver.

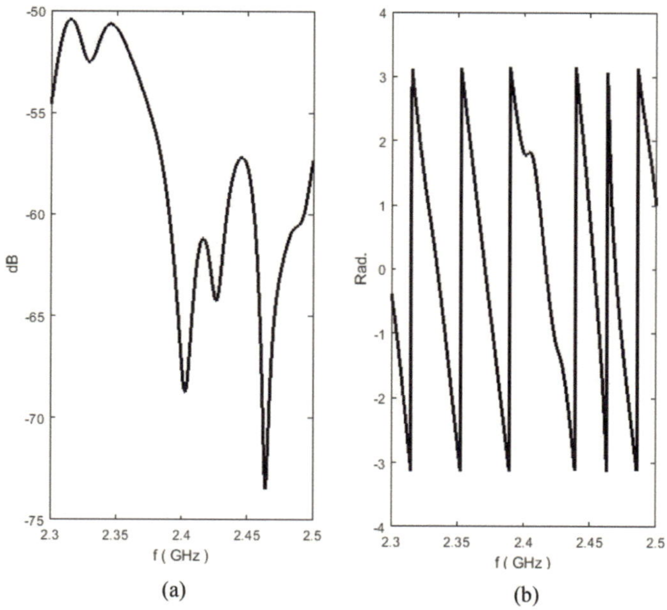

Figure 16. ANSYS Savant simulation result for coupling between the transmitter and receiver nodes for nonline of sight indoor communication scenario: (a) magnitude in dB and (b) phase in radians.

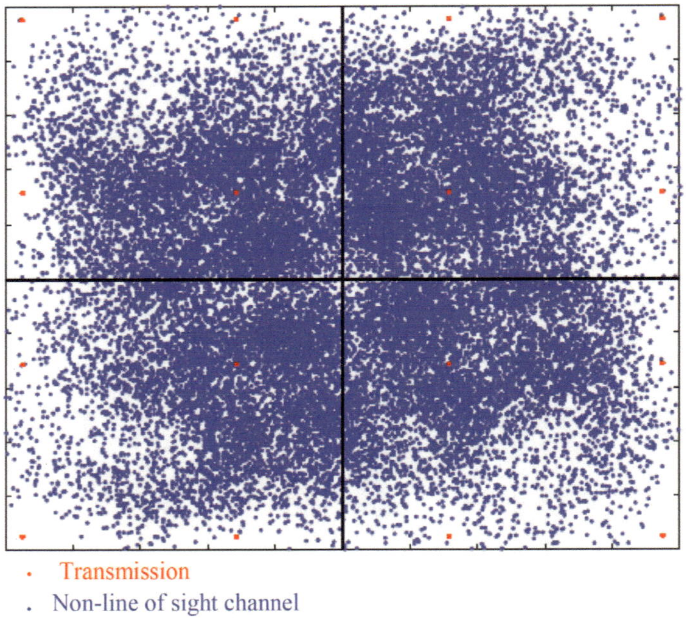

Figure 17. QAM-16 constellation plot at the receiver node for Case 2 (nonline of sight scenario).

5. Summary

In this chapter, some of the issues related to the antenna design and joint modeling of physical and communication layers for wireless body area networking were studied using ANSYS simulation tools. The design of a flexible patch antenna and evaluating its performance near the human body were investigated. Also, for the antenna size reduction, some of the related miniaturization techniques were reviewed. Moreover, a pervasive simulation and modeling idea was used to combine the physical layer simulation results with the communication (and networking) layers. The joint model was used to perform a case study and investigate how the wearable antenna's positioning relative to another wireless node can impact the communication between them for indoor applications.

Acknowledgements

The author would like to thank ANSYS Inc. for providing access to their simulation tools.

Author details

Mojtaba Fallahpour

Address all correspondence to: mfallahpour@ieee.org

ANSYS Inc., San Jose, CA, USA

References

[1] Movassaghi S, Abolhasan M, Lipman J, Smith D, Jamalipour A. Wireless body area networks: A survey. IEEE Communications Surveys & Tutorials. 2014;**16**(3):1658-1686

[2] Moghadam NN, Farhadi H, Bengtsson M. An energy efficient communication technique for medical implants/micro robots. IEEE International Symposium on Medical Information and Communication Technology (ISMICT'16); 2016

[3] Momenroodaki P, Haines W, Fromandi M, Popovic Z. Noninvasive internal body temperature tracking with near-field microwave radiometry. IEEE Transactions on Microwave Theory and Technique. 2018;**99**:1-11

[4] Momenroodaki P, Popović Z, Fallahpour M. Antenna probes for power reception from deep tissues for wearable microwave thermometry. In: 2017 IEEE International Sympo sium on Antennas and Propagation & USNC/URSI National Radio Science Meeting; San Diego, CA. 2017. pp. 573-574

[5] Fallahpour M, Zoughi R. Antenna miniaturization techniques: A review of topology- and material-based methods. IEEE Antennas and Propagation Magazine. Feb. 2018;**60**(1): 38-50

[6] Fallahpour M, Ghasr MT, Zoughi R. Miniaturized reconfigurable multiband antenna for multiradio wireless communication. IEEE Transactions on Antennas and Propagation. Dec. 2014;**62**(12):6049-6059

[7] Fallahpour M, Ghasr MT, Zoughi R. A multiband reconfigurable CPW-fed slot antenna. In: Proceedings of the 2012 IEEE International Symposium on Antennas and Propaga tion; Chicago, IL. 2012. pp. 1-2

[8] Chen ZN, Liu D, Nakano H, Qing X, Zwick T. Handbook of Antenna Technologies. Singapore: Springer; 2016

[9] www.ANSYS.com

[10] Chahat N, Zhadobov M, Sauleau R. Wearable textile patch antenna for BAN at 60 GHz. In: 7th European Conference on Antennas and Propagation (EuCAP); Gothenburg. 2013. pp. 217-219

[11] https://www.fcc.gov/general/radio-frequency-safety-0

[12] Medeiros CR, Costa JR, Fernandes CA. RFID reader antennas for tag detection in self-confined volumes at UHF. IEEE Antennas and Propagation Magazine. Apr. 2011;**53**(2): 39-50

[13] Amendola S, Milici S, Marrocco G. Performance of epidermal RFID dual-loop tag and on-skin retuning. IEEE Transactions on Antennas and Propagation. Aug. 2015;**63**(8): 3672-3680

[14] Velan S et al. Dual-band EBG integrated monopole antenna deploying fractal geometry for wearable applications. IEEE Antennas and Wireless Propagation Letters. 2015;**14**: 249-252

Chapter 4

Robust Optimal Power Distribution for Hyperthermia Cancer Treatment

Nafiseh Shariati, Dave Zachariah,
Johan Karlsson and Mats Bengtsson

Additional information is available at the end of the chapter

http://dx.doi.org/10.5772/intechopen.73281

Abstract

We consider an optimization problem for spatial power distribution generated by an array of transmitting elements. Using ultrasound hyperthermia cancer treatment as a motivating example, the signal design problem consists of optimizing the power distribution across the tumor and healthy tissue regions, respectively. The models used in the optimization problem are, however, invariably subject to errors. To combat such unknown model errors, we formulate a robust signal design framework that can take the uncertainty into account using a worst-case approach. This leads to a semi-infinite programming (SIP) robust design problem, which we reformulate as a tractable convex problem that potentially has a wider range of applications.

Keywords: power distribution, hyperthermia therapy, cancer treatment, robust transmission, optimization, MIMO

1. Introduction

Local hyperthermia is a noninvasive technique for cancer treatment, in which targeted body tissue is exposed to high temperatures to damage cancer cells, leaving surrounding tissue unharmed. This technique is used both to kill-off cancer cells in tumors and as a means to enhance other treatments such as radiotherapy and chemotherapy. Hyperthermia has the potential to treat many types of cancer, including sarcoma, melanoma, and cancers of the head and neck, brain, lung, esophagus, breast, bladder, rectum, liver, appendix, cervix, etc. [1–3].

Hyperthermia treatment planning involves modeling patient-specific tissue, using medical imaging techniques such as microwave, ultrasound, magnetic resonance or computed tomography, and calculating the spatial distribution of power deposited in the tissue to heat it [4]. There exist two major techniques to concentrate the power in a well-defined tumor region: electromagnetic and ultrasound, each with its own limitations. The drawback of electromagnetic microwaves is its poor penetration in biological tissue; while for ultrasound, the short acoustic wavelength renders the focal spot very small. Using signal design methods, however, one can improve the spatial power deposition generated by an array of acoustic transducers. Specifically, standard phased array techniques do not make use of combining a diversity of signals transmitted at each transducer. When this diversity is exploited, it is possible to dramatically improve the power distribution in the tumor tissue, thus improving the effectiveness of the method and reducing treatment time [5, 6]. Given a set of spatial coordinates that describe the tumor region and the healthy tissue, respectively, the transmitted waveforms can be designed to optimize the spatial power distribution while subject to certain design constraints.

One critical limitation, however, is the assumption of an ideal wave propagation model from the transducers to a given point in the tissue. Specifically, model mismatches may arise from hardware imperfections, tissue inhomogeneities, inaccurately specified propagation velocities, etc. Thus, the actual power distribution may differ substantially from the ideal one designed by an assumed model. This results in suboptimal clinical outcome due to loss of power in the tumor region and safety issues due to the possible damage of healthy tissue. These considerations motivate developing robust design schemes that take such unknown errors into account.

In this chapter, we derive a robust optimization method that only assumes the unknown model errors to be bounded. The power is then optimized with respect to "worst-case" model errors. By using a worst-case model, we provide an optimal signal design scheme that takes into account all possible, bounded model errors. Such a conservative approach is warranted in signal design for medical applications due to safety and health considerations. Our method further generalizes the approach in [5] by obviating the need to specify a fictitious tumor center point. The framework developed here has potential use in wider signal design applications where the resulting transmit power distributions are subject to model inaccuracies. More specifically, the design problem formulated in this chapter and the proposed robust scheme can be exploited to robustify the spatial power distribution for applications that an array equipped with multiple elements is used to emit waveforms in order to deliver power to an area of interest in a controlled manner.

The core of this study is built upon exploiting waveform diversity which has been introduced in multiple-input multiple-output (MIMO) radar literature [7], and later has been applied for local hyperthermia cancer treatment improvement in [5]. In the MIMO radar field, robustness studies have been carried out in different applications under varying design parameter uncertainties, cf., [8, 9]. Recently, in [10], we have studied the robustification of the waveform diversity methodology for MIMO radar applications. It should be highlighted that, in this chapter, a more generic problem formulation has been studied with respect to those of [10], where a new application area is considered to illustrate the performance of our proposed robust design. In the array processing literature, beamforming under array model errors has also spawned extensive work, cf., [11–14].

For hyperthermia therapy, the need for robust solutions when optimizing for phase and amplitude of conventional phased array has been investigated in [15], considering perfusion uncertainties, and in [16] considering dielectric uncertainties. The authors emphasize on the role of uncertainty in such designs (hyperthermia planning) since it influences the calculation of power distribution, and correspondingly temperature distribution.

The chapter is organized as follows: in Section 2, we describe the system model and the relevant variables. In Section 3, the signal design problem is presented. First, we consider the state-of-the-art method based on "waveform diversity" [5, 7, 17], then we generalize the design problem by introducing a deterministic and bounded set of possible model errors which results in an infinite number of constraints. Importantly, we show that this seemingly intractable problem can be equivalently formulated as a tractable convex optimization problem. In Section 4, we evaluate the design scheme. We evaluate the performance of our proposed robust power distribution scheme specifically for local hyperthermia breast cancer treatment. This example application is motivated by the alarming statistics pointing to breast cancer as one of the leading causes of death among women worldwide [18–20].[1] The case of no model mismatch is investigated first, and then the robust design scheme is applied, where its power distribution in the worst-case model is evaluated and compared to the nonrobust formulation.

Notation: Boldface (lower case) is used for column vectors, $\mathbf{x}$, and (upper case) for matrices, $\mathbf{X}$. $\|\mathbf{a}\|_{\mathbf{W}} \triangleq \sqrt{\mathbf{a}^H \mathbf{W} \mathbf{a}}$, where $\mathbf{W} > \mathbf{0}$. $\mathbf{x}^T$ and $\mathbf{x}^H$ denote transpose and Hermitian transpose, respectively. $\mathbf{R} \succeq \mathbf{0}$ signifies a positive semi-definite matrix and $\mathbf{R}^{1/2}$ signifies a matrix square-root, e.g., Hermitian. The set of complex numbers is denoted by $\mathcal{C}$.

Abbreviations: semi-infinite programming (SIP); multiple-input multiple-output (MIMO); semidefinite program (SDP); linear matrix inequality (LMI).

2. System model

We consider an array of M acoustic transducers to heat target points. These transducers are located at known positions $\boldsymbol{\theta}_m$, for $m = 1, 2, \ldots, M$, around the tissue at risk, cf., [5, 10]. We parameterize an arbitrary point in 3D space using Cartesian coordinates $\mathbf{r} = [x\, y\, z]^T$.

Let $x_m(n)$ denote the baseband representation of narrowband discrete-time signal transmitted at the mth transducer, at sample $n = 1, \ldots, N$. Then, the baseband signal received at a generic location $\mathbf{r}$ equals the superposition of signals from all M transducers, i.e.,

[1]Breast cancer is the most common cancer in the UK [18]. The risk of being diagnosed with breast cancer is 1 in 8 for women in the UK and US [18, 19]. Breast cancer is also stated to be a leading cause of cancer death in the less developed countries [20].

$$\begin{aligned} y(\mathbf{r},n) &= \sum_{m=1}^{M} a_m(\mathbf{r})x_m(n), \quad n=1,\dots,N \\ &= \mathbf{a}^H(\mathbf{r})\mathbf{x}(n), \quad n=1,\dots,N, \end{aligned} \tag{1}$$

where the mth signal is attenuated by a factor $a_m(\mathbf{r})$ which depends on the properties of the transducers, the carrier wave, and the tissue. This factor is modeled as

$$a_m(\mathbf{r}) = \frac{e^{-j2\pi f_c \tau_m(\mathbf{r})}}{\|\boldsymbol{\theta}_m - \mathbf{r}\|^{\frac{1}{2}}}, \tag{2}$$

where f_c is the carrier frequency, and $\tau_m(\mathbf{r}) = \frac{\|\boldsymbol{\theta}_m - \mathbf{r}\|}{c}$ is the required time for any signal to arrive at location $\mathbf{r}$ where c is the sound speed inside the tissue. Note that the root-squared term in the denominator of (2) represents the distance-dependent propagation attenuation of the acoustic waveforms. In (1), the narrowband signals are represented in vector form $\mathbf{x}(n) = [x_1(n)\dots x_m(n)\dots x_M(n)]^T \in \mathcal{C}^{M\times 1}$ and $\mathbf{a}(\mathbf{r}) \triangleq [a_1(\mathbf{r})\dots a_m(\mathbf{r})\dots a_M(\mathbf{r})]^T \in \mathcal{C}^{M\times 1}$ is the array steering vector as a function of $\mathbf{r}$.

At a generic location $\mathbf{r}$ in the tissue, the power of the transmitted signal, i.e., *the transmit beampattern*, is given by

$$p(\mathbf{r}) = \mathbb{E}\left\{|y(\mathbf{r},n)|^2\right\} = \mathbf{a}^H(\mathbf{r})\mathbf{R}\mathbf{a}(\mathbf{r}), \tag{3}$$

where

$$\mathbf{R} \triangleq \mathbb{E}\{\mathbf{x}(n)\mathbf{x}^H(n)\}$$

is the $M \times M$ covariance matrix of the signal $\mathbf{x}(n)$. As Eq. (3) suggests, the transmit beampattern is dependent on the waveform covariance matrix $\mathbf{R}$ and the array steering vector $\mathbf{a}(\mathbf{r})$. In the following, we analyze how one can form and control the beampattern by optimizing the covariance matrix $\mathbf{R}$, so as to heat up the tumor region of the tissue while keeping the power deposition in the healthy tissue minimal. In this work, we consider schemes which allow for the lowest possible power leakage to the healthy area.

Once an optimal covariance matrix $\mathbf{R}$ has been determined, the waveform signal $\mathbf{x}(n)$ can be synthesized accordingly. One simple approach is $\mathbf{x}(n) = \mathbf{R}^{1/2}\mathbf{w}(n)$, where $\mathbf{w}(n)$ is a sequence of independent random vectors with mean zero and covariance matrix $\mathbf{I}$. For detailed discussion see [21–23, Ch. 14].

A significant challenge to this approach, however, is that the *true* steering vector $\mathbf{a}(\mathbf{r})$ in (3) does not exactly match the model in (2) for a host of reasons: array calibration imperfections, variations in transducing elements, tissue inhomogeneities, inaccurately specified propagation velocity, etc. We will therefore consider the aforementioned design problem subject to model uncertainties in the array steering vector at any given point $\mathbf{r}$. We refer to this approach as robust waveform diversity.

3. Problem formulation

The waveform-diversity-based technique [5, 7, 10, 22, 24] have been used for designing beampatterns (3) subject to practical constraints. In general, we aim to control and shape the spatial power distribution at a set of target points while simultaneously minimizing power leakage in the remaining area. By exploiting a combination of different waveforms in (1), the degrees of freedom increase for optimizing the beampattern under constraints.

After reviewing the standard waveform diversity approach, we focus on the practical scenario where the assumed array steering vector model is subject to perturbations. In the subsequent section, the proposed robust technique is evaluated by numerical simulations, comparing the performance with and without robustified solution under perturbed steering vectors.

3.1. Waveform-Diversity-based Ultrasound System

In the MIMO radar literature, sidelobe minimization is a beampattern design problem that has been addressed by using the waveform diversity methodology, cf., [7, 21, 22, 24]. This design problem can be thought of as an optimization problem, where the probing waveforms covariance matrix $\mathbf{R}$ is the optimization variable to be chosen under positive semi-definiteness assumption and with a constraint on the total power. The waveform-diversity-based scheme for ultrasound system has been introduced and explained in detail in [5] based on the transmit beampattern design technique for MIMO radar systems [7, 24].

In the following, we consider the practical power constraint, where all array elements have the same power. Therefore, the covariance matrix $\mathbf{R}$ belongs to the following set $\mathcal{R}$:

$$\mathcal{R} \triangleq \left\{ \mathbf{R} | \mathbf{R} \succeq \mathbf{0}, R_{mm} = \frac{\gamma}{M}, m = 1, 2, \dots, M \right\}, \tag{4}$$

where γ is the total transmitted power and R_{mm} is the mth diagonal element of $\mathbf{R}$ corresponding to the power emitted by mth transducer. The healthy tissue and the tumor regions are represented by two sets of discrete control points $\mathbf{r}$:

$$\Omega_S = \{\mathbf{r}_1, \mathbf{r}_2, \dots, \mathbf{r}_{N_S}\} \tag{5}$$

$$\Omega_T = \{\mathbf{r}_1, \mathbf{r}_2, \dots, \mathbf{r}_{N_T}\}, \tag{6}$$

where N_S and N_T denote the number of points in the healthy tissue region and the tumor regions, respectively. Without loss of generality, let $\mathbf{r}_0$ be a representative point which is taken to be the center of the tumor region Ω_T. The objectives for this optimization problem can be summarized as follows: design the waveform covariance matrix $\mathbf{R}$ so as to

- maximize the gap between the power at the tumor center $\mathbf{r}_0$ and the power at the control points $\mathbf{r}$ in the healthy tissue region Ω_S;
- while guaranteeing a certain power level for control points $\mathbf{r}$ in the tumor region Ω_T.

Mathematically, this problem is formulated as (see [5])

$$\begin{aligned} \max_{\mathbf{R}, t} \quad & t \\ \text{s.t.} \quad & \mathbf{a}^H(\mathbf{r}_0)\mathbf{R}\mathbf{a}(\mathbf{r}_0) - \mathbf{a}^H(\mathbf{r})\mathbf{R}\mathbf{a}(\mathbf{r}) \geq t, \forall \mathbf{r} \in \Omega_S \\ & \mathbf{a}^H(\mathbf{r})\mathbf{R}\mathbf{a}(\mathbf{r}) \geq (1-\delta)\mathbf{a}^H(\mathbf{r}_0)\mathbf{R}\mathbf{a}(\mathbf{r}_0), \forall \mathbf{r} \in \Omega_T \\ & \mathbf{a}^H(\mathbf{r})\mathbf{R}\mathbf{a}(\mathbf{r}) \leq (1+\delta)\mathbf{a}^H(\mathbf{r}_0)\mathbf{R}\mathbf{a}(\mathbf{r}_0), \forall \mathbf{r} \in \Omega_T \\ & \mathbf{R} \in \mathcal{R} \end{aligned} \tag{7}$$

where t denotes the gap between the power at $\mathbf{r}_0$ and the power at the control points $\mathbf{r}$ in the healthy region Ω_S. The parameter δ is introduced here to control the required certain power level at the control points in the tumor region. For instance, if we set $\delta = 0.1$, then we aim for having power at the tumor region Ω_T to be within 10% of $p(\mathbf{r}_0)$, i.e., the power at the tumor center. This is an SDP problem which can be solved efficiently in polynomial time using any SDP solver, e.g., CVX [25, 26].

3.2. Robust waveform-diversity-based ultrasound system

The convex optimization problem (7) and consequently its optimal solution, i.e., the optimal covariance matrix $\mathbf{R}$, are functions of the steering vectors $\mathbf{a}(\mathbf{r})$. In practice, however, the assumed steering vector model used to optimize $\mathbf{R}$ is inaccurate. Hence, using *nominal* steering vectors $\hat{\mathbf{a}}(\mathbf{r})$ based on an ideal model, in lieu of the unknown *true* steering vectors $\mathbf{a}(\mathbf{r})$ in (7), may result in undesired beampatterns with low power at the tumor region and damaging power deposition in the healthy tissue region. Such health considerations in medical applications motivate an approach that is robust with respect to the worst-case model uncertainties.

In order to formulate the robust design problem mathematically, we parameterize the steering vector uncertainties as follows. Let the true steering vector for the transducer array be $\mathbf{a}(\mathbf{r}) = \hat{\mathbf{a}}(\mathbf{r}) + \tilde{\mathbf{a}}(\mathbf{r})$, where $\tilde{\mathbf{a}}(\mathbf{r})$ is an unknown perturbation from the nominal steering vector. The deterministic perturbation at any generic point $\mathbf{r}$ belongs to the uncertainty set $\mathcal{E}_{\mathbf{r}}$ that is bounded

$$\mathcal{E}_{\mathbf{r}} \triangleq \{\tilde{\mathbf{a}}(\mathbf{r}) \quad | \quad \|\tilde{\mathbf{a}}(\mathbf{r})\|_{\mathbf{W}}^2 \leq \varepsilon_{\mathbf{r}}\}, \tag{8}$$

where $\mathbf{W}$ is a $M \times M$ diagonal weight matrix with positive elements. The weight matrix $\mathbf{W}$ can be derived based on the type of uncertainty. Using $\mathbf{W}$, the set $\mathcal{E}_{\mathbf{r}}$ indicates an ellipsoidal region. The bound $\epsilon_{\mathbf{r}}$ for the set can be a constant or a function of $\mathbf{r}$, i.e., $\epsilon_{\mathbf{r}} = f(\mathbf{r})$. This set enables parameterization of element-wise uncertainties in the nominal steering vector $\hat{\mathbf{a}}(\mathbf{r})$ at each $\mathbf{r}$.

Besides this consideration, we generalize the problem formulation (7) further by setting a uniform bound (power level) P across the tumor region Ω_T as an optimization variable to which the power of all the control points in the healthy region Ω_S are compared. This is in contrast to (7) and the robust formulation in [10], where the power levels of all the healthy grid points Ω_S are compared with the power of only a single reference point at fictitious tumor center $\mathbf{r}_0$. There is no need to limit our problem to a single point as a reference power level. Rather, the desired tightness of the power level across Ω_T is specified by the parameter $0 \leq \delta < 1$. This generalization also improves the efficiency when it comes to solving the robust design problem.

With these considerations, the robust beampattern design problem can be formulated as

$$\begin{aligned} \max_{\mathbf{R},\, t,\, P} \quad & t \quad \text{subject to} \\ & P - (\hat{\mathbf{a}}(\mathbf{r}) + \tilde{\mathbf{a}}(\mathbf{r}))^H \mathbf{R} (\hat{\mathbf{a}}(\mathbf{r}) + \tilde{\mathbf{a}}(\mathbf{r})) \geq t, \forall \tilde{\mathbf{a}}(\mathbf{r}) \in \mathcal{E}_{\mathbf{r}}, \mathbf{r} \in \Omega_S \\ & (\hat{\mathbf{a}}(\mathbf{r}) + \tilde{\mathbf{a}}(\mathbf{r}))^H \mathbf{R} (\hat{\mathbf{a}}(\mathbf{r}) + \tilde{\mathbf{a}}(\mathbf{r})) \geq (1-\delta)P, \forall \tilde{\mathbf{a}}(\mathbf{r}) \in \mathcal{E}_{\mathbf{r}}, \mathbf{r} \in \Omega_T \\ & (\hat{\mathbf{a}}(\mathbf{r}) + \tilde{\mathbf{a}}(\mathbf{r}))^H \mathbf{R} (\hat{\mathbf{a}}(\mathbf{r}) + \tilde{\mathbf{a}}(\mathbf{r})) \leq (1+\delta)P, \forall \tilde{\mathbf{a}}(\mathbf{r}) \in \mathcal{E}_{\mathbf{r}}, \mathbf{r} \in \Omega_T \\ & \mathbf{R} \in \mathcal{R}, \end{aligned} \tag{9}$$

where t is the gap between the desired power levels set across Ω_T and power deposition in the healthy tissue Ω_S, similar to (7). Note that we take into account every possible perturbation $\tilde{\mathbf{a}}(\mathbf{r}) \in \mathcal{E}_{\mathbf{r}}$.

In contrast to the optimization problem (7), which is a tractable convex problem, the robust problem (9) is an SIP problem. For a given $\mathbf{R}$ in (9), there are infinite number of constraints in terms of $\tilde{\mathbf{a}}(\mathbf{r})$ to satisfy which makes the problem non-trivial. However, in the following theorem, extending the approach in [10], we reformulate the robust power deposition problem as a convex SDP problem whose solution is the optimally robust covariance matrix.

Theorem 1. *The robust power deposition for an M-element transducer array with the probing signal covariance matrix* $\mathbf{R} \in \mathcal{R}$ *and the perturbation vector* $\tilde{\mathbf{a}}(\mathbf{r}) \in \mathcal{E}_{\mathbf{r}}$, *i.e., the solution of* (9), *is given as a solution to the following SDP problem*

$$\begin{aligned} \max_{\mathbf{R},\, t,\, P,\, \beta_i,\, \beta_{j,1},\, \beta_{j,2}} \quad & t \quad \text{subject to} \\ \Omega_S: & \begin{bmatrix} \beta_i \mathbf{W} - \mathbf{R} & -\mathbf{R}\hat{\mathbf{a}}(\mathbf{r}_i) \\ -\hat{\mathbf{a}}(\mathbf{r}_i)^H \mathbf{R} & P - t - \hat{\mathbf{a}}(\mathbf{r}_i)^H \mathbf{R} \hat{\mathbf{a}}(\mathbf{r}_i) - \beta_i \varepsilon_{\mathbf{r}_i} \end{bmatrix} \succeq \mathbf{0}, \\ \Omega_T: & \begin{bmatrix} \beta_{j,1} \mathbf{W} + \mathbf{R} & \mathbf{R}\hat{\mathbf{a}}(\mathbf{r}_j) \\ \hat{\mathbf{a}}(\mathbf{r}_j)^H \mathbf{R} & \hat{\mathbf{a}}(\mathbf{r}_j)^H \mathbf{R} \hat{\mathbf{a}}(\mathbf{r}_j) - (1-\delta)P - \beta_{j,1} \varepsilon_{\mathbf{r}_j} \end{bmatrix} \succeq \mathbf{0}, \\ \Omega_T: & \begin{bmatrix} \beta_{j,2} \mathbf{W} - \mathbf{R} & -\mathbf{R}\hat{\mathbf{a}}(\mathbf{r}_j) \\ -\hat{\mathbf{a}}(\mathbf{r}_j)^H \mathbf{R} & (1+\delta)P - \hat{\mathbf{a}}(\mathbf{r}_j)^H \mathbf{R} \hat{\mathbf{a}}(\mathbf{r}_j) - \beta_{j,2} \varepsilon_{\mathbf{r}_j} \end{bmatrix} \succeq \mathbf{0}, \\ & \mathbf{R} \in \mathcal{R}, \beta_i, \beta_{j,1}, \beta_{j,2} \geq 0, i = 1, \ldots, N_S, j = 1, \ldots, N_T. \end{aligned} \tag{10}$$

Proof: See Appendix A.

Observe that the notations Ω_S and Ω_T indicate that the corresponding linear matrix inequalities (LMIs) should be satisfied for the points $\mathbf{r}_i \in \Omega_S$ and $\mathbf{r}_j \in \Omega_T$, respectively. Note that the robust SDP problem in this chapter, which is stated in Theorem 1, can be solved more efficiently than the SDP problem in [10] since the matrices **R** and **W** in the current formulation have half of the size of the matrices involved in the latter problem. This occurs due to the generalization of the robust problem by using the uniform power level as a benchmark.

Note that other robust problems with similar objectives can also be addressed using the above approach which are outlined in the following subsection.

3.3. Alternative robust formulations

Similar robust problems to that of (9) can be formulated in many different ways. For example, by restricting the power level outside the tumor in a weighted fashion.

$$\begin{aligned}
&\min_{t, R} t \quad \text{subject to} \\
&(\widehat{\mathbf{a}}(\mathbf{r}) + \tilde{\mathbf{a}}(\mathbf{r}))^H R(\widehat{\mathbf{a}}(\mathbf{r}) + \tilde{\mathbf{a}}(\mathbf{r})) \le tw(\mathbf{r}), \forall \tilde{\mathbf{a}}(\mathbf{r}) \in \mathcal{E}_{\mathbf{r}}, \mathbf{r} \in \Omega_S \\
&(\widehat{\mathbf{a}}(\mathbf{r}) + \tilde{\mathbf{a}}(\mathbf{r}))^H R(\widehat{\mathbf{a}}(\mathbf{r}) + \tilde{\mathbf{a}}(\mathbf{r})) \ge (1-\delta)P, \forall \tilde{\mathbf{a}}(\mathbf{r}) \in \mathcal{E}_{\mathbf{r}}, \mathbf{r} \in \Omega_T \\
&(\widehat{\mathbf{a}}(\mathbf{r}) + \tilde{\mathbf{a}}(\mathbf{r}))^H R(\widehat{\mathbf{a}}(\mathbf{r}) + \tilde{\mathbf{a}}(\mathbf{r})) \le (1+\delta)P, \forall \tilde{\mathbf{a}}(\mathbf{r}) \in \mathcal{E}_{\mathbf{r}}, \mathbf{r} \in \Omega_T \\
&R \in \mathcal{R}
\end{aligned} \tag{11}$$

where P, δ are fixed and $w(\mathbf{r})$ is a weighting function constructed, e.g., so that the energy bound close to the tumor is less restrictive.

One could also construct problems that minimize the sum of the energy in the non-tumor area, where $t(\mathbf{r})$ denotes the energy at $\mathbf{r}$:

$$\begin{aligned}
&\min_{t(\mathbf{r}), R} \sum_{\mathbf{r} \in \Omega_S} t(\mathbf{r}) \quad \text{subject to} \\
&(\widehat{\mathbf{a}}(\mathbf{r}) + \tilde{\mathbf{a}}(\mathbf{r}))^H R(\widehat{\mathbf{a}}(\mathbf{r}) + \tilde{\mathbf{a}}(\mathbf{r})) \le t(\mathbf{r}), \forall \tilde{\mathbf{a}}(\mathbf{r}) \in \mathcal{E}_{\mathbf{r}}, \mathbf{r} \in \Omega_S \\
&(\widehat{\mathbf{a}}(\mathbf{r}) + \tilde{\mathbf{a}}(\mathbf{r}))^H R(\widehat{\mathbf{a}}(\mathbf{r}) + \tilde{\mathbf{a}}(\mathbf{r})) \ge (1-\delta)P, \forall \tilde{\mathbf{a}}(\mathbf{r}) \in \mathcal{E}_{\mathbf{r}}, \mathbf{r} \in \Omega_T \\
&(\widehat{\mathbf{a}}(\mathbf{r}) + \tilde{\mathbf{a}}(\mathbf{r}))^H R(\widehat{\mathbf{a}}(\mathbf{r}) + \tilde{\mathbf{a}}(\mathbf{r})) \le (1+\delta)P, \forall \tilde{\mathbf{a}}(\mathbf{r}) \in \mathcal{E}_{\mathbf{r}}, \mathbf{r} \in \Omega_T \\
&R \in \mathcal{R}.
\end{aligned} \tag{12}$$

Both of the alternative formulations described above can be addressed following the steps derived in Appendix A by using $\mathcal{S}$-lemma, since we are still dealing with quadratic constraints.

In the next section, we illustrate the reference performance of a nominal scenario where the steering vectors are perfectly known. Then, we observe how much power can leak to the healthy tissue and cause damages when subject to uncertain steering vectors. Finally, we evaluate the proposed robust scheme in terms of improving the power deposition along our stated design goals.

4. Numerical results

To illustrate the performance of the proposed robust scheme, we consider a 2D model of the organ at risk. Here, similar to [5], we focus on the ultrasonic hyperthermia treatment for breast cancer where a 10-cm-diameter semicircle is assumed to model breast tissues with a 16-mm-diameter tumor embedded inside. The tumor center is located at $\mathbf{r}_0 = [0 \quad 34]^T$ mm. **Figure 1** shows this schematic model. We consider a curvilinear array with $M = 51$ acoustic transducers and half wavelength element spacing. Acoustic waveforms used to excite the array have the carrier frequency of 500 kHz. The acoustic wave speed for the breast tissue is considered as 1500 m/s.

To characterize (discretize) the healthy tissue region Ω_S and the tumor region Ω_T, two grid sets with the spacing 4 mm are considered. For optimization, a rectangular surface of the dimension 64×42 in mm is assumed symmetric around the tumor to model the healthy region Ω_S, while the grid points belonging to the circular tumor region are excluded from this surface and they model Ω_T. Overall, 174 and 13 number of control points are considered to characterize Ω_S and Ω_T in order to optimize the array beampattern.

The total transmitted power is constrained to $\gamma = 1$. For simplicity, the uncertainty set $\mathcal{E}_\mathbf{r}$ is modeled with $\mathbf{W} = \mathbf{I}_M$ and with $\boldsymbol{\epsilon}_\mathbf{r} \equiv \boldsymbol{\epsilon}$ for all $\mathbf{r}$, where $\boldsymbol{\epsilon} = 0.25$. Furthermore, the tightness of the desired power level in the across tumor region, δ, is set to 0.7. Note that for the small values of δ and/or large values of $\boldsymbol{\epsilon}$, the problem may turn infeasible. In general, the feasibility of the problem depends on the value of the tightness bound δ relative to the size of the existing uncertainty in the system, i.e., the volume of the uncertainty set $\boldsymbol{\epsilon}$, and the number of grid points N_S and N_T used to control the beampattern at the area of interest. When δ is too small, the desired power level across Ω_T is close to uniform and there may not exist enough degrees of freedom for the design problem to have a solution.

For reference, the optimal covariance matrix when no uncertainty is taken into account, $\mathbf{R}_{nr}$, is obtained by solving problem (9) using only nominal steering vectors $\hat{\mathbf{a}}(\mathbf{r})$, i.e., $\tilde{\mathbf{a}}(\mathbf{r}) \equiv \mathbf{0}$. The optimal robust covariance matrix, denoted $\mathbf{R}^\star$, is obtained by solving (10), where $\tilde{\mathbf{a}}(\mathbf{r}) \in \mathcal{E}_\mathbf{r}$. For

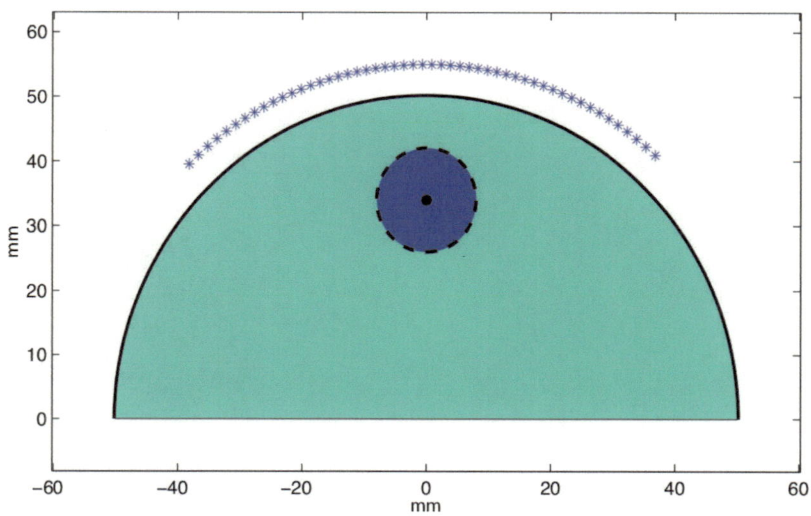

Figure 1. A schematic 2-D breast model with a 16-mm embedded tumor at $(0, 34)$ as a reference geometry. A curvilinear ultrasonic array with 51 transducers is located near to the organ at risk. The ultrasonic array is used for hyperthermia treatment.

performance evaluation, we consider the power deposition in the tissue under the worst-case perturbations of the steering vectors. This scenario provides a lower bound to the achievable performances of all steering vector perturbations $\tilde{\mathbf{a}}(\mathbf{r})$, which belong to the deterministic uncertainty set $\mathcal{E}_{\mathbf{r}}$. In other words, for the points $\mathbf{r}$ in the healthy region Ω_S, the worst-case performance is rendered by the steering vectors which provide the highest power; whereas, for the points $\mathbf{r}$ in the tumor region Ω_T, those steering vectors which attain the lowest power are the ones which contribute in the worst-case performance. They are collectively referred to as the *worst steering vectors*. Therefore, for a given $\mathbf{R}$, either $\mathbf{R}_{nr}$ or $\mathbf{R}^{\star}$, the worst steering vectors for the control points $\mathbf{r}$ in Ω_S and Ω_T are obtained by maximizing and minimizing the transmit beampattern (3), respectively. Observe that finding the worst steering vectors for the points in the tumor region Ω_T equals solving the following convex minimization problem at each $\mathbf{r} \in \Omega_T$, i.e.,

$$\min_{\|\tilde{\mathbf{a}}(\mathbf{r})\|^2 \leq \varepsilon} \quad (\widehat{\mathbf{a}}(\mathbf{r}) + \tilde{\mathbf{a}}(\mathbf{r}))^H \mathbf{R} (\widehat{\mathbf{a}}(\mathbf{r}) + \tilde{\mathbf{a}}(\mathbf{r})) \tag{13}$$

using CVX [25, 26]. Whereas, for finding the worst steering vectors for the points in the healthy region Ω_S, we obtain a local optimum for the following nonconvex maximization problem at each $\mathbf{r} \in \Omega_S$, i.e.,

$$\max_{\|\tilde{\mathbf{a}}(\mathbf{r})\|^2 \leq \varepsilon} \quad (\widehat{\mathbf{a}}(\mathbf{r}) + \tilde{\mathbf{a}}(\mathbf{r}))^H \mathbf{R} (\widehat{\mathbf{a}}(\mathbf{r}) + \tilde{\mathbf{a}}(\mathbf{r})), \tag{14}$$

using semidefinite relaxation techniques from [27].

We evaluate the designed beampatterns (3) plotting the spatial power distribution in decibel scale, i.e., $20\log_{10}(p(\mathbf{r}))$. Two different scenarios are considered, namely *nominal* and *perturbed*, to evaluate the proposed robust power distribution scheme for the ultrasonic array. In the first scenario, nominal, we assume that the array steering vectors are precisely modeled, i.e., $\tilde{\mathbf{a}}(\mathbf{r}) = \mathbf{0}$. In **Figure 2**, the beampattern generated by the array is plotted for the nominal

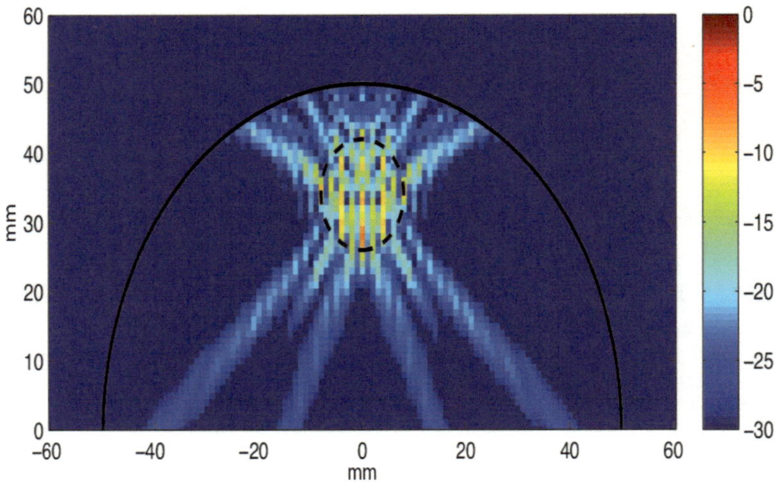

Figure 2. Power distribution (transmit beampattern in dB) for the nominal scenario, i.e., using $\mathbf{R}_{nr}$ and $\tilde{\mathbf{a}}(\mathbf{r}) \equiv 0$.

scenario. This figure represents how power is spatially distributed over the organ at risk in an idealistic situation. Here, the covariance matrix of the waveforms is optimized under the assumption that the steering vectors are accurately modeled by (2), and the performance is evaluated using exactly the same steering vectors without any perturbations. The power is noticeably concentrated in the tumor region and importantly the power in the healthy tissue is several decibels lower.

In the second scenario, perturbed, the idealistic assumptions are relaxed and model uncertainties and imperfections are taken into account. The second scenario represents the case, where the true steering vectors are perturbed versions of the nominal steering vectors $\widehat{\mathbf{a}}(\mathbf{r})$, i.e., the true steering vector equals $\widehat{\mathbf{a}}(\mathbf{r}) + \tilde{\mathbf{a}}(\mathbf{r})$ where $\tilde{\mathbf{a}}(\mathbf{r}) \in \mathcal{E}_{\mathbf{r}}$. The perturbation vectors $\tilde{\mathbf{a}}(\mathbf{r})$ are unknown but deterministically bounded. In the following, we illustrate the worst-case

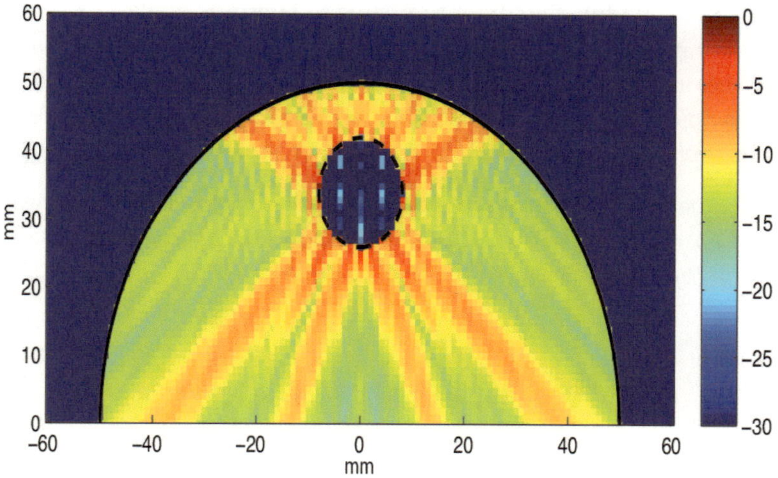

Figure 3. Power distribution (transmit beampattern in dB) for the perturbed scenario, i.e., using $\mathbf{R}_{nr}$ and $\tilde{\mathbf{a}}(\mathbf{r}) \in \mathcal{E}_{\mathbf{r}}$.

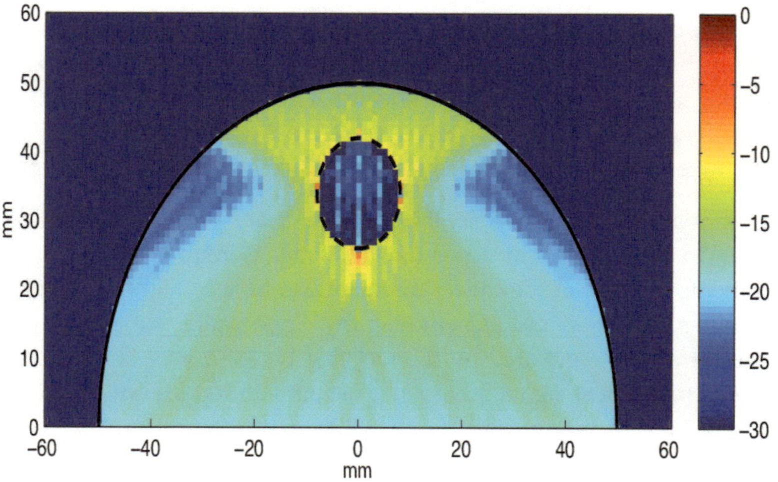

Figure 4. Power distribution (transmit beampattern in dB) for the perturbed scenario, i.e., using $\mathbf{R}^{\star}$ and $\tilde{\mathbf{a}}(\mathbf{r}) \in \mathcal{E}_{\mathbf{r}}$.

Scenarios	Ω_T	Ω_S
Nominal, $\mathbf{R}_0$	−16.54	−29.78
Perturbed, $\mathbf{R}_0$	−36.40	−11.69
Perturbed, $\mathbf{R}^\star$	−27.17	−17.43

Table 1. Average power for different regions.

performance, i.e., using the worst steering vectors to calculate the power distribution at each point. We start by illustrating the beampattern for the nonrobust covariance matrix $\mathbf{R}_{nr}$ under the worst steering vectors. **Figure 3** shows how steering vector errors can degrade the array performance. Notice that in the worst-case, there is a substantial power leakage that occurs in the healthy tissue surrounding the tumor compared to **Figure 2**. While, in **Figure 4**, the robust optimal covariance matrix $\mathbf{R}^\star$, i.e., the solution to (10), is used to calculate the power for the worst steering vectors. Comparing **Figures 3** and **4**, we see that by taking model uncertainties into account it is possible to obtain a noticeable increase in power in the tumor region for the worst-case, and importantly, dramatic reductions of power deposited in the healthy tissue.

To finalize the numerical analysis, we provide a quantitative description for the performance of our proposed scheme summarized in **Table 1**. It shows the average power calculated in dB received at the tumor region Ω_T and at the healthy region Ω_S.

5. Conclusion

The robust transmit signal design for optimizing spatial power distribution of a multi-antenna array is investigated. A robustness analysis is carried out to combat against inevitable uncertainty in model parameters which results in performance degradation. Such degradation occurs in practice quite often due to relying on imperfect prior and designs based upon them. Particularly, in this chapter, the transmit signal design is based on exploiting the waveform diversity property, but where errors in the array steering vector are taken into account. These errors are modeled as belonging to a deterministic set defined by a weighted norm. Then, the resulting robust signal covariance optimization problem with infinite number of constraints is translated to a convex problem which can be solved efficiently by using the $\mathcal{S}$-procedure.

Designs that are robust with respect to the worst-case are particularly vital in biomedical applications due to health risks and possible damage. Herein, we have focused on local hyperthermia therapy as one of the cancer treatments to be used either individually or along with other treatments such as radio/chemotherapy. Specifically, we consider hyperthermia treatment of breast cancer motivated by the fact that breast cancer is a major global health concern. The proposed robust signal design scheme aims to reduce unwanted power leakage into the healthy tissue surrounding the tumor while guaranteeing certain power level in the tumor region itself.

We should emphasize on the fact that the robust design problem formulation and the analysis carried out herein yielding to the robust waveforms are general enough to be exploited whenever spatial power distribution is a concern to be addressed in real world scenarios dealing with uncertainties, e.g., for radar applications.

Numerical examples representing different scenarios are given to illustrate the performance of the proposed scheme for hyperthermia therapy. We have observed significant power leakage into the healthy tissue that can occur if the design is based on uncertain model parameters. Importantly, we have shown how such damaging power deposition can be avoided using the proposed robust design for optimal spatial power distribution.

Acknowledgements

The authors would like to acknowledge Prof. Jian Li for providing an implementation of examples from [4].

A. Appendix

A.1. Proof of Theorem 1

We start the proof by first stating the $\mathcal{S}$-Procedure lemma, which helps us to turn the optimization problem (6) with infinitely many quadratic constraints into a convex problem with finite number of LMIs.

Lemma 1. *($\mathcal{S}$-Procedure ([28], Lemma 4.1): Let $f_k(\mathbf{x}) : \mathbb{C}^n \rightarrow \mathbb{R}$, $k = 0, 1$, be defined as $f_k(\mathbf{x}) = \mathbf{x}^H \mathbf{A}_k \mathbf{x} + 2\mathrm{Re}\{\mathbf{b}_k^H \mathbf{x}\} + c_k$, where $\mathbf{A}_k = \mathbf{A}_k^H \in \mathbb{C}^{n\times n}$, $\mathbf{b}_k \in \mathbb{C}^n$, and $c_k \in \mathbb{R}$. Then, the statement (implication) $f_0(\mathbf{x}) \geq 0$ for all $\mathbf{x} \in \mathbb{C}^n$ such that $f_1(\mathbf{x}) \geq 0$ holds if and only if there exists $\beta \geq 0$ such that*[2]

$$\begin{bmatrix} \mathbf{A}_0 & \mathbf{b}_0 \\ \mathbf{b}_0^H & c_0 \end{bmatrix} - \beta \begin{bmatrix} \mathbf{A}_1 & \mathbf{b}_1 \\ \mathbf{b}_1^H & c_1 \end{bmatrix} \succeq 0, \tag{15}$$

if there exists a point $\widehat{\mathbf{x}}$ with $f_1(\widehat{\mathbf{x}}) > 0$.

The constraints in the optimization problem (9) can be rewritten as the following functions of $\tilde{\mathbf{a}}(\mathbf{r})$ for $\mathbf{r} \in \Omega_S$ and $\mathbf{r} \in \Omega_T$. For notation simplicity, we only specify the set from which the control points are drawn, and we also drop $\mathbf{r}$.

[2]Note that $\mathcal{S}$-Procedure is lossless in complex space for the case of at most two constraints [29].

$$\Omega_S : \begin{cases} f_0 = -\tilde{\mathbf{a}}^H\mathbf{R}\tilde{\mathbf{a}} - 2\mathrm{Re}\left(\hat{\mathbf{a}}^H\mathbf{R}\tilde{\mathbf{a}}\right) - \hat{\mathbf{a}}^H\mathbf{R}\hat{\mathbf{a}} - t + P \geq 0 \\ f_1 = -\tilde{\mathbf{a}}^H\mathbf{W}\tilde{\mathbf{a}} + \varepsilon_\mathbf{r} \geq 0 \end{cases}$$

$$\Omega_T : \begin{cases} f_0 = \tilde{\mathbf{a}}H\mathbf{R}\tilde{\mathbf{a}} + 2\mathrm{Re}\left(\hat{\mathbf{a}}^H\mathbf{R}\tilde{\mathbf{a}}\right) + \hat{\mathbf{a}}^H\mathbf{R}\hat{\mathbf{a}} - (1-\delta)P \geq 0 \\ f_1 = -\tilde{\mathbf{a}}^H\mathbf{W}\tilde{\mathbf{a}} + \varepsilon_\mathbf{r} \geq 0 \end{cases}$$

$$\Omega_T : \begin{cases} f_0 = -\tilde{\mathbf{a}}H\mathbf{R}\tilde{\mathbf{a}} - 2\mathrm{Re}\left(\hat{\mathbf{a}}^H\mathbf{R}\tilde{\mathbf{a}}\right) - \hat{\mathbf{a}}^H\mathbf{R}\hat{\mathbf{a}} + (1+\delta)P \geq 0 \\ f_1 = -\tilde{\mathbf{a}}^H\mathbf{W}\tilde{\mathbf{a}} + \varepsilon_\mathbf{r} \geq 0 \end{cases} \tag{16}$$

Now, according to the $\mathcal{S}$-Procedure lemma, each pair of the quadratic constraints above is replaced with an LMI for each grid points in the pre-defined sets. In other words, all these quadratic constraints are satisfied simultaneously if we find β_i for $i = 1, \ldots, N_S$, $\beta_{j,1}$ and $\beta_{j,2}$ for $j = 1, \ldots, N_T$, for which the mentioned LMIs in Theorem 1 holds. Thus, the problem boils down to the SDP problem (10) with $2N_T + N_S$ LMIs of the size $(M+1) \times (M+1)$ as the constraints. □

Author details

Nafiseh Shariati[1]*, Dave Zachariah[2], Johan Karlsson[3] and Mats Bengtsson[4]

*Address all correspondence to: nafiseh.shariati@ericsson.com

1 Ericsson Research, Stockholm, Sweden

2 Department of Information Technology, Division of Systems and Control, Uppsala University, Uppsala, Sweden

3 Department of Mathematics, KTH Royal Institute of Technology, Stockholm, Sweden

4 Division of Information Science and Engineering, KTH Royal Institute of Technology, Stockholm, Sweden

References

[1] Falk M, Issels R. Hyperthermia in oncology. International Journal of Hyperthermia. 2001; **17**(1):1-18

[2] van der Zee J. Heating the patient: A promising approach? Annals of Oncology. 2002; **13**(8):1173-1184

[3] Wust P, Hildebrandt B, Sreenivasa G, Rau B, Gellermann J, Riess H, Felix R, Schlag P. Hyperthermia in combined treatment of cancer. The Lancet Oncology. 2002;**3**(8):487-497

[4] Paulides MM, Stauffer PR, Neufeld E, Maccarini PF, Kyriakou A, Canters RAM, Diederich CJ, Bakker JF, Van Rhoon GC. Simulation techniques in hyperthermia treatment planning. International Journal of Hyperthermia. 2013;**29**(4):346-357

[5] Guo B, Li J. Waveform diversity based ultrasound system for hyperthermia treatment of breast cancer. IEEE Transactions on Biomedical Engineering. 2008;**55**(2):822-826

[6] Jennings MR, McGough RJ. Improving conformal tumour heating by adaptively removing control points from waveform diversity beamforming calculations: A simulation study. International Journal of Hyperthermia. 2010;**26**(7):710-724

[7] Stoica P, Li J, Xie Y. On probing signal design for MIMO radar. IEEE Transactions on Signal Processing. 2007;**55**(8):4151-4161

[8] Yang Y, Blum RS. Minimax robust MIMO radar waveform design. IEEE Journal of Selected Topics in Signal Processing. 2007;**1**(1):147-155

[9] Grossi E, Lops M, Venturino L. Robust waveform design for MIMO radars. IEEE Transactions on Signal Processing. 2011;**59**(7):3262-3271

[10] Shariati N, Zachariah D, Bengtsson M. Minimum sidelobe beampattern design for MIMO radar systems: A robust approach. In: IEEE International Conference on Acoustics, Speech and Signal Processing (ICASSP); May 2014. pp. 5312-5316

[11] Li J, Stoica P, Wang ZS. Doubly constrained robust capon beamformer. IEEE Transactions on Signal Processing. 2004;**52**(9):2407-2423

[12] Yan S, Hovem J. Array pattern synthesis with robustness against manifold vectors uncertainty. IEEE Journal of Oceanic Engineering. 2008;**33**(4):405-413

[13] Kim SJ, Magnani A, Mutapcic A, Boyd SP, Luo ZQ. Robust beamforming via worst-case SINR maximization. IEEE Transactions on Signal Processing. 2008;**56**(4):1539-1547

[14] Khabbazibasmenj A, Vorobyov SA, Hassanien A. Robust adaptive beamforming based on steering vector estimation with as little as possible prior information. IEEE Transactions on Signal Processing. 2012;**60**(6):2974-2987

[15] de Greef M, Kok HP, Correia D, Bel A, Crezee J. Optimization in hyperthermia treatment planning: The impact of tissue perfusion uncertainty. Medical Physics. 2010;**37**(9):4540-4550

[16] de Greef M, Kok H, Correia D, Bel A, Crezee J. Uncertainty in hyperthermia treatment planning: The need for robust system design. Physics in Medicine and Biology. 2011; **56**(11):3233-3250

[17] Li J, Stoica P. MIMO radar—Diversity means superiority. In: MIMO Radar Signal Processing. NJ: John Wiley and Sons; 2009

[18] Cancer Research UK. Breast Cancer Key Facts [Online]. Available from: http://www.cancerresearchuk.org

[19] American Cancer Society. Breast Cancer [Online]. Available from: http://www.cancer.org/

[20] International Agency for Research on Cancer. Press Releases [Online]. Available from: http://www.iarc.fr/en/media-centre/pr/2013

[21] Stoica P, Li J, Zhu X, Guo B. Waveform synthesis for diversity-based transmit beampattern design. In: IEEE 14th Workshop on Statistical Signal Processing (SSP '07); 2007. pp. 473-477

[22] Fuhrmann DR, San Antonio G. Transmit beamforming for MIMO radar systems using signal cross-correlation. IEEE Transactions on Aerospace and Electronic Systems. 2008; **44**(1):171-186

[23] He H, Li J, Stoica P. Waveform Design for Active Sensing Systems—A Computational Approach. UK: Cambridge University Press; 2012

[24] Fuhrmann DR, San Antonio G. Transmit beamforming for MIMO radar systems using partial signal correlation. In: IEEE 38th Asilomar Conference on Signals, Systems and Computers; Vol. 1; 2004. pp. 295-299

[25] Grant M, Boyd S. CVX: Matlab Software for Disciplined Convex Programming, Version 2.0 Beta. 2013. http://cvxr.com/cvx

[26] Graph implementations for nonsmooth convex programs. In: Blondel V, Boyd S, Kimura H, editors. Recent Advances in Learning and Control. Lecture Notes in Control and Information Sciences. London, UK: Springer-Verlag Limited; 2008. pp. 95-110. http://stanford.edu/~boyd/graph dcp.html

[27] Beck A, Eldar YC. Strong duality in nonconvex quadratic optimization with two quadratic constraints. SIAM Journal on Optimization. 2006;**17**(3):844-860

[28] Beck A. Convexity properties associated with nonconvex quadratic matrix functions and applications to quadratic programming. Journal of Optimization Theory and Applications. 2009;**142**(1):1-29

[29] Jönsson UT. A Lecture on the S-Procedure. 2001. http://www.math.kth.se/optsyst/forskning/forskarutbildning/SF3849/Lecture

Chapter 5

Gait-Based Smart Pairing System for Personal Wearable Devices

Weitao Xu and Guohao Lan

Additional information is available at the end of the chapter

http://dx.doi.org/10.5772/intechopen.74195

Abstract

With the rapid development of embedded technology and mobile computing, we have seen a growing number of Internet of Things (IoT) devices on the market. As the number of wearable devices belonging to the same user increases rapidly, secure pairing between legitimate devices becomes an important research problem. In this chapter, we propose the first gait-based shared key generation system that assists two devices to generate a common secure key by exploiting the user's unique walking pattern. The system is based on the fact that sensors on different positions of the same user exhibit similar accelerometer signal when the user is walking. Therefore, the acceleration can be used as a shared secret information to generate a common key on different devices independently. Our experimental results show that the key generated by two independent devices on the same body is able to achieve 100% bit agreement rate. The proposed key generation protocol can establish a 128-bit key in 5 s (about 10 steps) with entropy varying from 0.93 to 1. We also find that the proposed scheme can run in real time on modern smartphone and require low system cost.

Keywords: wearable devices, authentication, key generation, system implementation, evaluation

1. Introduction

With recent advances in wireless sensor networks and embedded computing technologies, wearable and implantable devices such as smartphone, smartwatch and pacemaker have become increasingly popular and play significant roles in our daily lives. For users, it is of potentially great value to associate a personal device with another device in a spontaneous manner, i.e. without need for pre-configuration between two legitimate devices. Pairing devices can be used for the purpose of short-lived interactions, for example, file transfer and synchronization, or aimed at longer lived pairing, for example, pairing a smartphone with accessories.

The wireless nature of the communication between devices gives rise to problems of authentication and security [1]. **Figure 1** presents an example of on-body devices with potential adversaries. An adversary can listen to the communication between legitimate devices and eavesdrop private information. Traditional security mechanisms rely on cryptographic keys to support integrity and confidentiality services. Usually, two parties will first establish a common key, and then use the key to encrypt/decrypt subsequent communications between these two devices. In a dynamic mobile environment, mobile devices need to establish point-to-point association frequently. However, it is difficult to ensure the availability of a certificate authority or a key management center. Therefore, it is necessary to have alternative method for key distribution between mobile devices without resorting to a fixed infrastructure.

In current mobile systems, this is achieved by key exchange methods, which are either manual (e.g. typing in the key in a keypad) or exploit key-exchange algorithms. For the first case, a common mechanism for peer device authentication is personal identification number (PIN) code entry by the user into the involved devices [2]. Another example is that the user needs to make sure two devices show the same PIN code on the display when pairing devices using Bluetooth.

However, a primary requirement for human-involved authentication is ease of use and can interact with another device without much user intervention. Such methods offer a reasonably secure way of establishing a common key, but can only be acceptable for occasional use. The number of pairing between wearable devices can be expected to grow considerably as mobile

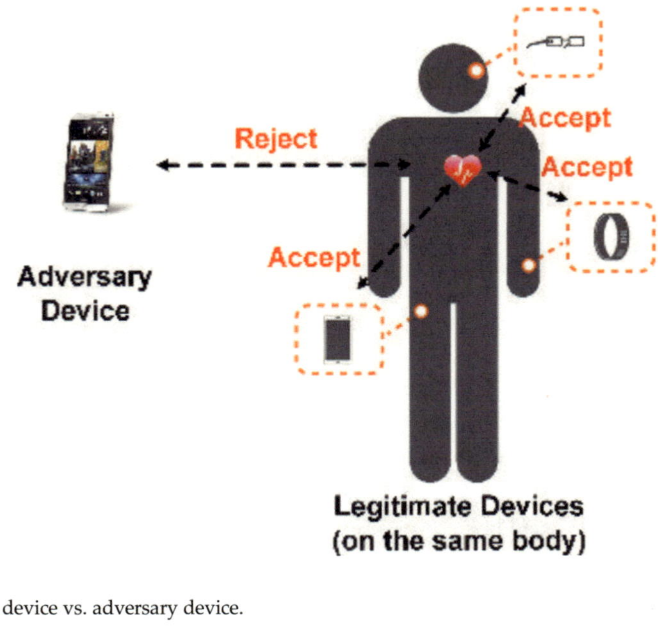

Figure 1. Legitimate device vs. adversary device.

devices are becoming increasingly pervasive. Therefore, the human-involved authentication method is undesirable when users seek to engage in fast and short-lived authentications frequently. To address the problem of pairing devices frequently, one can save the secure key on the device and use it next time. However, this method cannot ensure the security of the key because the stored key can be stolen. On the other hand, due to the small form factor and user interface (UI) of wearable devices, such method is not well suitable because wearable devices are not assumed to include screen and keyboard, e.g. pacemaker and health monitor. For the key-exchange algorithm, a common key exchange method is Diffie-Hellman (DH) protocol which is used to distribute a symmetric key between two parties [3]. However, the premise of DH protocol is that two devices to be paired together are legitimate devices. It cannot be used to distinguish adversary device with legitimate devices.

In this chapter, we propose and implement a shared secret key generation protocol for smart wearable devices based on gait. Gait refers to a person's manner of walking [4]. The intuition of the proposed key generation protocol is that devices on the same body experience similar signals when the user is walking. Therefore, the similar signals can be used to generate a shared secret key between legitimate devices. The proposed protocol provides an intuitive, unobtrusive method to pair wearable devices when they are on the same body. To the best of our knowledge, this is the first work to generate a key for wearable devices based on gait. The main contributions of this paper are two-fold:

1. Shared key generation protocol: We present a novel, lightweight key generation protocol for wearable devices based on gait signals. We experimentally demonstrate that the keys generated on two separate wearable devices on the same body can achieve a 100% bit agreement rate. The proposed key generation protocol is able to generate a 128-bit key with entropy varying from 0.93 to 1 by walking 5 s (≈10 steps).

2. Implementation: We implement the proposed key generation protocol on modern smartphone. We report system overhead such as processing time and power consumption, and demonstrate the feasibility of the proposed protocol for use in contemporary wearable devices.

The rest of the chapter is organized as follows. We first introduce system model in Section 2. Then we specify the shared key generation protocol in Section 3. We evaluate the performance of the proposed key generation protocol in Section 4 and implement the system in Section 5. Finally, Section 6 concludes the chapter.

2. System model

We envision the use of the proposed system primarily for pairing wearable and implantable devices such as smartphone, smartwatch and pacemaker. **Figure 2** illustrates a typical user model: a user wants to read private health information from pacemaker (Bob) through a smart watch (Alice). He walks several steps, and then Alice and Bob generate a shared secret key by exploiting the gait signals. The key is then used to encrypt/decrypt the messages between two parties.

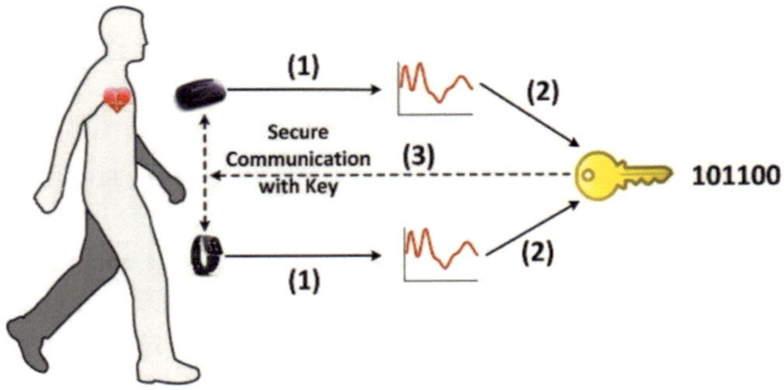

Figure 2. System model.

3. Design overview

In this section, we will provide an overview of the proposed scheme. **Figure 3** illustrates the flowchart of the key generation protocol. Suppose Alice (smartphone) wants to read data from Bob (pacemaker). Alice first broadcasts a *REQ* request to Bob. After receiving *REQ*, Bob replies a *ACK* message back to Alice. Then Alice and Bob start to collect data and follow the steps shown in **Figure 3** to generate a shared secret key. Finally, the key is used to secure the subsequent communication between Alice and Bob. The key component of the proposed scheme consists of the following two steps:

1. Signal processing. Signal processing consists of two steps: temporal alignment and spatial alignment. Temporal alignment is used to synchronize acceleration samples at Alice and Bob. Spatial alignment is used to transform the acceleration data to the same coordinate system to facilitate key generation.

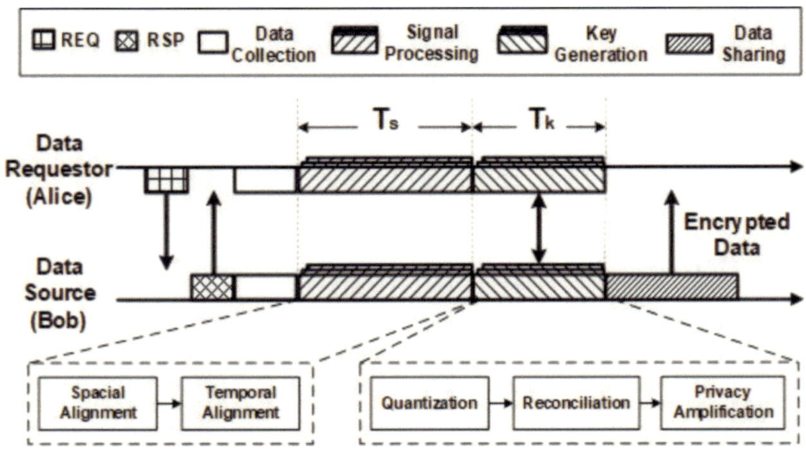

Figure 3. System flowchart.

2. Key generation. The key generation phase is composed of three parts: quantization, reconciliation and privacy amplification. In quantization stage, Alice and Bob convert their observed information into bits. In reconciliation stage, Alice and Bob exchange some information to agree on the same bit string. Finally, privacy amplification technique is used to diminish the partial information eavesdropped by Eve.

In the following sections, we will describe design details of each component in turn.

3.1. Signal processing

In this section, we describe spatial alignment which is used to transform the original acceleration data into the same coordinate system and temporal alignment which addresses the problem of synchronization.

3.1.1. Spatial alignment

Walking is inherently a three-dimensional movement. 3D acceleration data cannot be directly used for key generation because they are recorded at different locations and orientations. We address this problem by transforming accelerometer data of different devices to the same reference coordinate system. **Figure 4** shows the definition of device coordinate system, the global coordinate system, and the body reference coordinate system. We define the world coordinate system by North, East and the Earth gravity (−G). The device coordinate system is defined as (X, Y, Z). The user plane of motion is defined as forward-sideway plane that is perpendicular to gravity. Sideway points to the right side of the body's forward direction. Take smart watch as an example, assume the linear acceleration signals along three orthogonal directions of smart watch are Acc_x, Acc_y and Acc_z, respectively, the linear acceleration in the body reference system can be calculated by the following equation:where Acc_X′, Acc_Y′ and Acc_Z′ are linear acceleration along gravity direction, forward direction and sideway direction in the body reference system. *R* is the rotation matrix from the device coordinate

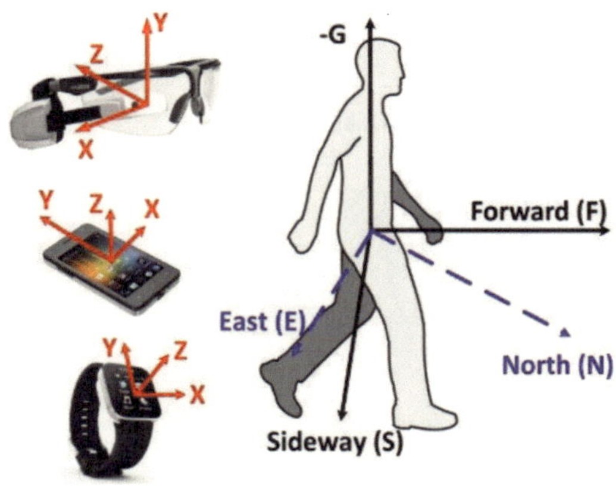

Figure 4. The different coordinate systems: the coordinate system of device is defined as (X, Y, Z). The world coordinate system is defined as (E, N, −G). The user plane of motion is the forward-sideway (F-S) plane, which is the plane perpendicular to gravity.

system to the world coordinate system and can be obtained by the method in [5]. The authors in [5] proposed a method to reliably and accurately estimate the user orientation in different environments at arbitrary phone positions and orientations. Their proposed method first fuses different phone inertial sensors to obtain the phone orientation and then applies principal component analysis (PCA) to improve the final accuracy. After obtaining the acceleration in body coordinate system, we use Acc_X′, Acc_Y′ and Acc_Z′ for key generation.

$$\begin{pmatrix} Acc\_X' \\ Acc\_Y' \\ Acc\_Z' \end{pmatrix} = R \begin{pmatrix} Acc\_x \\ Acc\_y \\ Acc\_z \end{pmatrix} \quad (1)$$

3.1.2. *Temporal alignment*

Temporal synchronization is necessary because different devices sample acceleration values independently. We adopt an event-based mechanism in which devices detect the time point of a heel-strike event, and use this event to trigger data collection. This method is based on the fact that the acceleration data along gravity direction reach the peak simultaneously when the foot touches the ground, and time delays in signal transmission through the body are negligible. In order to detect this event, we apply a low-pass filter on acceleration data Acc_X′ to reduce noise. The cut-off frequency is 3 Hz as we find the normal step frequency lies between 1.6–2.8 Hz [6]. Then the local peaks are detected to indicate heel-strike events as we can see from **Figure 5**.

The proposed method eliminates the requirement of explicit synchronization as heel-strike events can be detected locally at each device without communication. When Alice receives a *ACK* message from Bob, they both reach an agreement to record acceleration data from the next *i*-th heel-strike event and stop recording at the subsequent *j*-th event. Then the acceleration samples are processed by spatial alignment to the same coordinate system.

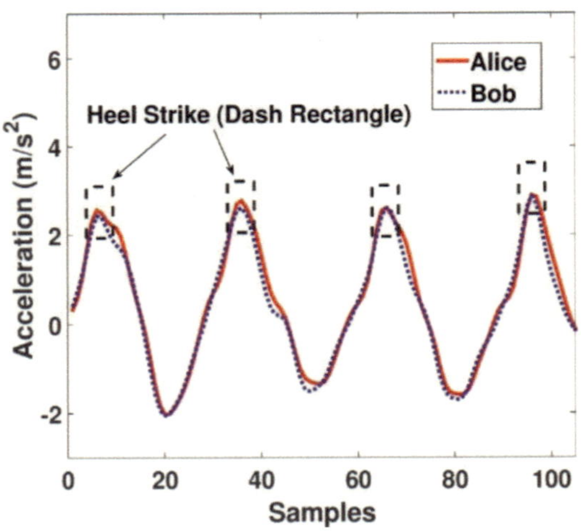

Figure 5. The peak along gravity direction indicates a heel strike on the ground.

http://dx.doi.org/10.5772/intechopen.74195

3.2. Key generation

3.2.1. Quantization

Our goal is to extract exactly the same cryptographic key if and only if two devices are on the same body. **Figure 6** plots the acceleration of two legitimate devices and an adversary device in three directions. Due to the fact that acceleration values of two devices on the same body are not identical as shown in **Figure 6**, the key generation algorithm must have the ability to map even similar sequences to the same key and less similarity to different keys. The key generation method is applied on two legitimate devices separately.

After signal alignment, we obtain acceleration values along three directions: Acc_X′, Acc_Y′ and Acc_Z′. To generate keys, we perform low-pass filtering and quantization for the acceleration values in these three directions independently. As the first step, we use a low-pass filter to filter out environmental noise. The cutoff frequency is chosen as 10 Hz as the useful frequency of human motion lies below 10 Hz. After filtering, the acceleration values are normalized to have zero mean and unit length to eliminate the impact of different positions. Bits are obtained by applying the bit generation approach in [7, 8]. In the proposed system, we segment the acceleration sequence with a moving window with no overlap (window size $W = 10$). We then calculate two thresholds $q+$ and $q-$ within each window:

$$q+ = u + \alpha * \delta, \quad q- = u - \alpha * \delta \tag{2}$$

where u and δ are the mean and standard deviation of acceleration values in a window. After obtaining $q+$ and $q-$, we generate bits by the following rule: the acceleration values which are > q + are encoded as bit 1, and values that are < q_- are encoded as bit 0. Finally, we combine the bits generated from each window together to form a bit string. **Figure 7** illustrates the quantization process in a window in detail.

After the above steps, we obtain three separate bit strings K_G, K_F, K_S. We concatenate these three bit strings together to form the initial key for Alice K_Alice = [K_G, K_F,K_S]. On Bob's side, he will perform the same quantization process to get K_Bob.

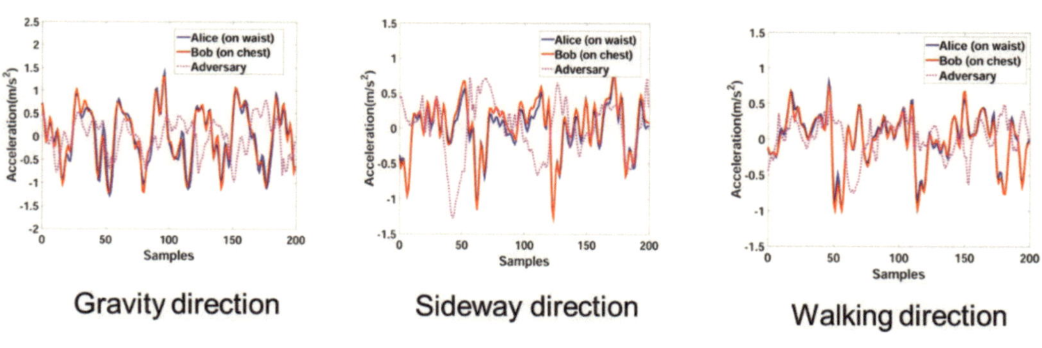

Figure 6. Acceleration along three directions.

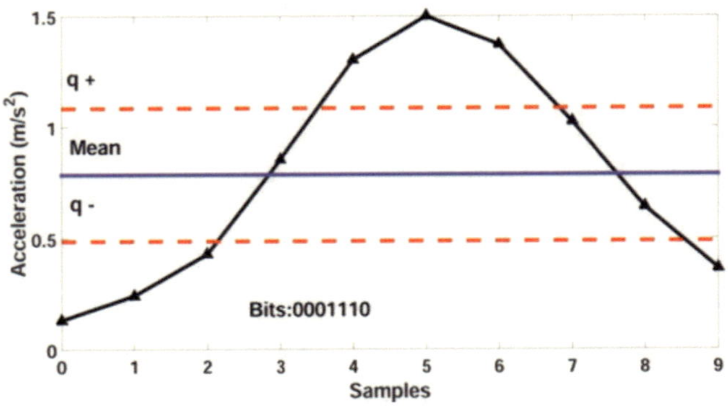

Figure 7. Quantization process.

3.2.2. *Reconciliation process*

After key generation, we often get K_Alice≈K_Bob in practice because of noise. In this section, we describe reconciliation process which is used to correct the mismatches between Alice and Bob. The main reason causing mismatches is that the samples discarded during quantization at Alice's side may be different from Bob's side. In order to correct the mismatches, they are required to exchange their sequence of sample indexes during reconciliation process. In this step, only the bits corresponding to common sample indexes are reserved by Alice and Bob to obtain the common key. For example, let us assume Alice and Bob each has 10 measurements in a window. After key generation, Alice obtains "01100" and Bob yields "0110". The length of these two keys is not required to be same because they may discard different number of acceleration samples during quantization. If we assume Alice generates bits at positions 1, 3, 5, 6 and 9, respectively. She sends L_Alice = [1, 3, 5, 6, 9] to Bob. Bob checks his own position information and finds the bits are generated at positions 1, 2, 5 and 9. He sends L_Bob = [1, 2, 5, 9] back to Alice. Then they use the bits at positions 1, 5 and 9 to generate the same key as K_Alice' = K_Bob' = "010."

3.2.3. *Privacy amplification process*

Because walking is a repetitive activity, different steps may have high correlation, thus decreasing the randomness of the key. This problem can be addressed by privacy amplification process. In the proposed system, we use XOR function to achieve this goal. Specifically, we interleave the bit streams from three directions in time sequence and segment the concatenated keys into small windows with no overlap. We then perform XOR operation on two consecutive windows together to obtain the final key which are denoted by K_Alice" and K_Bob".

Another function of privacy amplification is that it diminishes the partial information revealed to Eve. Because in the reconciliation stage, Alice and Bob exchange messages over an authenticated public channel and the publicly exchanged messages reveal a certain amount of information about the bit strings to Eve. Note that other privacy amplification methods such as universal hash [9] can be employed to further enhance the randomness of the concatenated key. We refer the reader to [9] for more details.

http://dx.doi.org/10.5772/intechopen.74195

4. Performance evaluation

In this section, we present the evaluation results. The aims of the evaluation are twofold: (1) to evaluate the impact and performance of different parameters such as the window size (W), α in quantization process, sampling frequency (F_s); (2) to evaluate the performance of different components in the system which includes reconciliation process and privacy amplification.

4.1. Data acquisition

We collected a set of accelerometer data from 20 subjects (14 males and 6 females) wearing smart devices on different locations of their body. As can be seen from **Figure 8**, the body positions involved in the data collection include head, chest, waist and wrist. These positions represent the common locations of mobile devices such as smartwatch and medical sensors (e.g. pacemaker). During the data acquisition, the sampling rate of all smart wearable devices is 100 Hz.

During data acquisition, the participants were asked to wear mobile devices as shown in **Figure 8** and walk for about 5 minutes in their normal speed (0.7–1.1 m/s). We collect data from both indoor and outdoor environments to capture different terrains in real-world scenarios. It is worth mentioning that we do not consider the influence of different days or different walking speeds

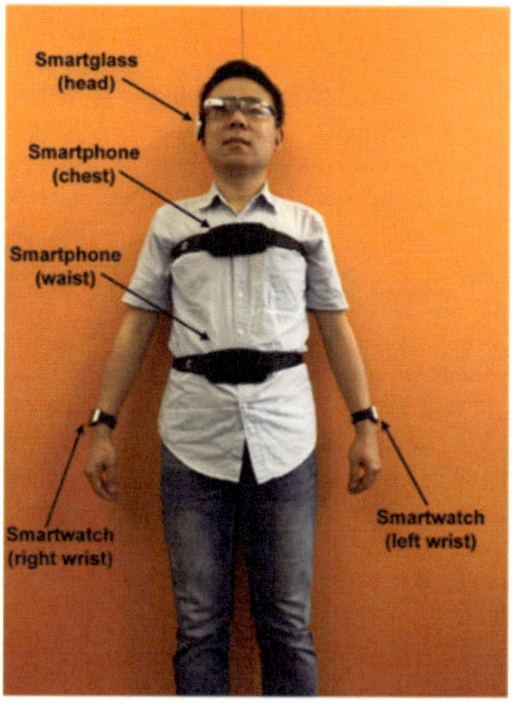

Figure 8. Data acquisition.

(slow, normal and fast) because all the devices worn by the subject are measuring the same gait signal simultaneously, which is different from the data collection requirement in the study of gait recognition [10]. The detected peaks that indicate heel strikes are used to synchronize acceleration samples recorded on different wearable devices and segment steps. For each device attached on one subject, we segment the acceleration sequences into small windows based on heel-strike points. In this experiment, each window contains 10 steps. Then these windows are passed to the system to generate final keys and evaluate the following metrics.

Three metrics are selected to quantitatively evaluate the performance:

- **Bit agreement rate**. Bit agreement rate denotes the percentage of matching bits in keys generated by two parties. This metric evaluates the potential that two parties (either two legitimate devices or a legitimate and an adversary device) can generate the same key.
- **Bit rate.** Bit rate denotes the number of bits generated in unit time, measured in bits per second (bps). This metric evaluates how fast the system can generate a secret key.
- **Entropy.** Entropy denotes randomness in generated keys. This metric measures the amount of information contains in each bit.

To evaluate the influence of different parameters on the system performance, we first conduct a systematic exhaustive search to find the optimal combination. We vary the respective parameters within a dedicated range, i.e. $F\_s = 10, 20, 30, 50, 100$, $\alpha = 0, 0.1, \ldots, 1$, and $W = 5, 10, \ldots, 50$. After this step, we find the best parameters combination is F_s = 30, $\alpha = 0.8$ and $W = 10$. Then we take turns to evaluate the influence of each parameter on system performance by setting the other two parameters to the optimal value.

As mentioned above, each subject has acceleration samples recorded from five different body parts. For each body part of one subject, we compute the bit agreement rate of legitimate devices by using keys generated from other locations on the same body. We show the results of the average values and 95% confidence level of the performance metrics (bit agreement rate and bit rate).

4.2. Influence of sampling rate

In this experiment, we evaluate the influence of different sampling rate by downsampling F_s from 100 to 50 Hz, 30, 20 and 10 Hz, respectively. The impact of F_s on bit rate and bit agreement rate are plotted in **Figure 9**, respectively. We find that sampling rate has a negative impact on the agreement rate between legitimate devices. After looking into the data, we find this is because a higher sampling rate is able to record more acceleration values during the same time window and thus increase bit rate; however, it reduces bit agreement as a higher sampling rate captures acceleration variation more precisely which results in more mismatches between legitimate devices.

4.3. Influence of parameter α

The parameter α in quantization phase determines the trade-off between agreement rate and bit rate. In this experiment, we will evaluate the influence of α. As we can see from **Figure 10**,

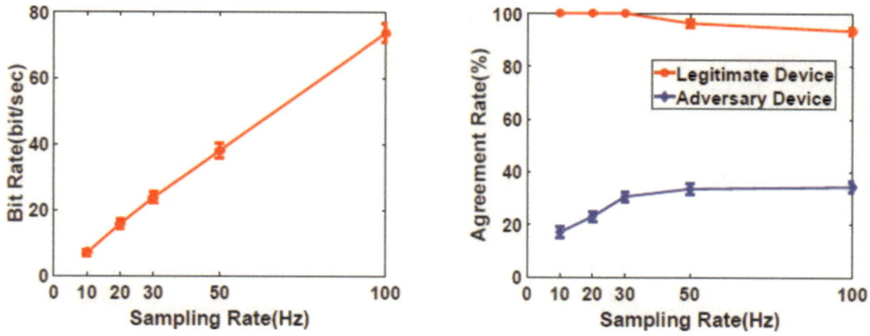

Figure 9. Influence of sampling rate.

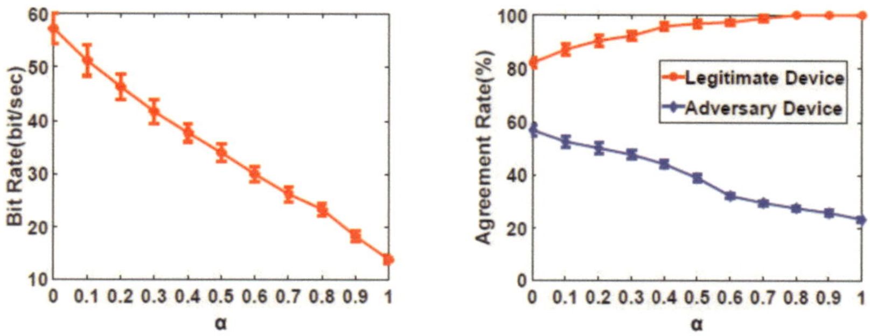

Figure 10. Impact of α.

the bit rate drops when α increases. This is because the parameter α in Eq. (2) determines the guard band which affects the inclusion or exclusion of acceleration samples. A larger α means we will discard more acceleration samples. This will reduce the bit rate. On the other hand, as we can see from **Figure 10**, the bit agreement rate increases with the growth of α because more mismatches are excluded. In the meantime, we observe that parameter α has inverse impact on agreement rate for an adversary device. This is because more samples are discarded for quantization at all the devices when α increases. Therefore, the legitimate devices know the index numbers used and they exchange the index list during reconciliation, so the agreement rate increases. However, for an attacker, she does not know which samples are kept because the signal values itself are different from that of legitimate devices, the remaining bits after discarding more acceleration measurements in quantization will have less bit agreement rate.

In addition to sampling rate and α, we also evaluated the influence of window size in the proposed system. We found that the moving window size W does not have much influence on the system performance and we set the moving window size to 10 for the proposed system.

4.4. Influence of reconciliation process

As described in Section 3.2.2, reconciliation process is necessary because it is used to reduce the mismatches between two parties. **Figure 11** shows the influence of reconciliation process on the bit rate and agreement rate. We can see a significant improvement in bit agreement rate

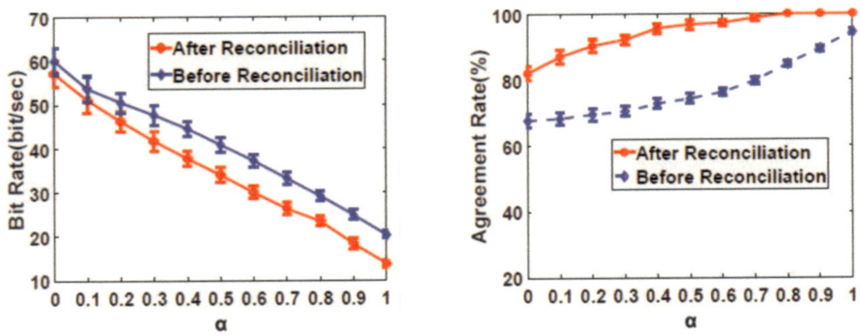

Figure 11. Influence of reconciliation.

after employing reconciliation approach. However, we also notice that the drawback of reconciliation approach used in our system is that it will reduce bit rate. Recall that the main goal of our system is to generate the same key; therefore, reconciliation is a necessary part of the proposed key extraction system.

4.5. Impact of privacy amplification

As mentioned in Section 3.2.3, privacy amplification is used to improve the randomness of the final key. In this experiment, we investigate if the XOR function in privacy amplification achieves this goal. **Figure 12** compares the entropy of the final key before and after privacy amplification. We find that the distribution of entropy is closer to 1 after XOR operation. We also notice that the entropy of the final keys varies from 0.93 to 1 which suggests that the proposed key generation protocol can generate secret keys with good entropy. It is worth mentioning that one disadvantage of using XOR function is that the bit rate will be reduced by a factor of 2 because we XOR two consecutive windows together. From the results in **Figure 11**, we find that the final bit rate can still reach 26 bit/sec after reconciliation and privacy amplification process. State-of-the-art cryptographic algorithms such as AES require a key

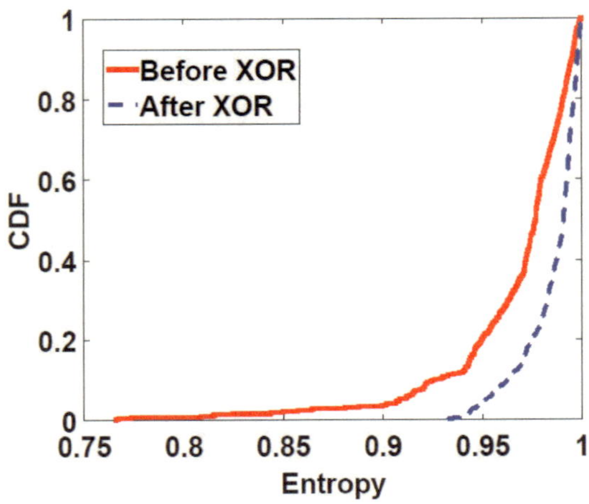

Figure 12. Impact of privacy amplification.

NIST test	p-values
Frequency	0.606072
FFT test	0.562699
Longest run	0.027173
Linear complexity	0.386887
Block frequency	0.984496
Cumulative sums	0.974180
Approximate entropy	0.995898
Nonoverlapping template	0.302941

Table 1. NIST test results.

length with at least 128 bits; therefore, our method takes about 5 s to generate a secure key (about 10 steps).

4.6. Evaluation of key randomness

The generated keys will be used for encryption and decryption; therefore, we need to guarantee that the generated keys are random. In this experiment, we apply the NIST suite of statistical tests to evaluate the randomness of the final keys generated from our dataset. The final results of NIST statistical test are p-values of different random test processes. If p-values are greater than 0.01, it indicates the bit string is generated by a random process. Otherwise, if p-values are below 0.01, the key is not random. From **Table 1**, we can see that the p-values are all greater than 1% which indicates the generated keys from our method are random.

5. System implementation

In order to demonstrate the feasibility of the proposed key generation protocol on mobile devices, we have prototyped the proposed scheme on Motorola Moto E2, a state-of-the-art mobile phone. The complete key generation scheme is implemented in Java. The sampling rate of accelerometer is set as 30 Hz, and Bluetooth low energy (BLE) functionality is employed for wireless communication. BLE is designed to provide significantly lower power consumption for devices with low power requirements, such as pacemaker. Therefore, BLE is well suited for the proposed key generation protocol. Moreover, devices working under BLE broadcasting mode do not need to be paired together beforehand.

BLE is designed to provide significantly lower power consumption for devices with low power requirements. It introduces a new feature called peripheral mode, in which the data source can advertise and publish data without requiring to pair with the data requestor beforehand. BLE peripheral mode is designed for devices with resource-constraint and need to publish new data frequently. Therefore, we run the system in peripheral mode and advertise the data using broadcast packets. Bob organizes its data using Generic Attribute Profile (GATT) and encrypts

	Computation time (ms)	Energy consumption(mJ)
Signal processing	108.3	72.7
Key generation	208.1	12.7
AES encryption	0.2	0.1
AES decryption	0.2	0.1
Total	316.8	85.6

Table 2. System overhead measured on Moto E2 smartphone.

the data to publish by AES. All the devices nearby including adversaries can receive the broadcast advertisements and read the public-available data from Bob. However, only Alice on the same body can generate the same key for data decryption. In this way, the private data is protected from reading by unauthorized devices.

We implement our protocol on two Moto E2 smartphones and use one of them to simulate pacemaker (Bob), the other one is used as smartphone (Alice) to request data from pacemaker. Both Alice and Bob work under BLE broadcasting mode. The main interface of Alice has a UI button that can be pressed by a user to trigger pairing process. After a user presses the start button on Alice, Alice and Bob follow the steps presented in **Figure 3** to generate a shared secret key. If the length of the final key is greater than 128, only the first 128 bits are considered. After obtaining a 128-bit length cryptographic key, Bob encrypts the heart rate measurement (simulated measurement) by Advanced Encryption Standard (AES) and broadcast the encrypted message. Although several nearby devices including adversaries can listen to the broadcast packets, only Alice can generate the same key and decrypt the messages.

Table 2 presents the system overhead (computation time and energy consumption) of our system on Moto E2. The computation time and energy consumption are computed by averaging the results from 50 trials. The computation time is obtained from the console of Android studio. The energy consumption is profiled by $E = PT$, where P is the average power and T is the running time of the profiled component. The average power $P = Current * Voltage$, where the *Current* and *Voltage* of the battery is obtained via Android APIs. The results in **Table 2** show that the execution of the two stages in the protocol: signal processing and key generation take an average time of 108.3 and 208.1 ms, respectively. When the scheme is fully employed, the computation time and energy consumption are 316.8 ms and 85.6 mJ, respectively. Note that heel-strike detection is applied on the continuous acceleration samples to detect heel-strike events. Therefore, the processing time and energy consumption are not applicable in **Table 2**. These results demonstrate the proposed key generation protocol has a low system overhead and can run in real time on modern mobile devices.

6. Conclusion

In this chapter, we propose and implement a key generation protocol that exploits the acceleration data produced by walking to establish a common cryptographic key between two wearable devices. Our protocol obtains a security advantage from the fact that different people have distinctive walking styles. We performed extensive experiments to evaluate the performance of our proposed system and demonstrate that the proposed key generation protocol is able to establish a 128-bit length key in about 5 s (about 10 steps). We also prototyped the proposed scheme on Motorola E2 smartphone to demonstrate the feasibility of our system on mobile devices.

Author details

Weitao Xu* and Guohao Lan

*Address all correspondence to: w.t.xu@unsw.edu.au

School of Computer Science and Engineering, University of New South Wales, Sydney, Australia

References

[1] Stajano F, Anderson R. The resurrecting duckling: Security issues in ad-hoc wireless networks. In: Proceedings of the 7th International Workshop in Security Protocols, Lecture Notes in Computer Science. London, UK: Springer-Verlag; 1999. http://www.cl.cam.ac.uk/fms27/duckling

[2] Gehrmann C, Mitchell CJ, Nyberg K. Manual authentication for wireless devices. RSA Cryptobytes. 2004;**7**(1):29-37

[3] Die W, Hellman ME. New directions in cryptography. IEEE Transactions on Information Theory. 1976;**22**(6):644-654

[4] Gafurov D, Snekkenes E, Buvarp TE. Robustness of biometric gait authentication against impersonation attack. In: Proceedings of on the Move to Meaningful Internet Systems 2006 (OTM 2006 Workshops). Berlin, Heidelberg: Springer; 2006. pp. 479-488

[5] Mohssen N, Momtaz R, Aly H, Youssef M. It's the human that matters: Accurate user orientation estimation for mobile computing applications. In: Proceedings of the 11th International Conference on Mobile and Ubiquitous Systems: Computing, Networking and Services (MOBIQUITOUS). ICST (Institute for Computer Sciences Social-Informatics and Telecommunications Engineering), London, United Kingdom; 2014. pp. 70-79

[6] Murray MP. Gait as a total pattern of movement: Including a bibliography on gait. American Journal of Physical Medicine & Rehabilitation. 1967;**46**(1):290-333

[7] Revadigar G, Javali C, Hu W, Jha S. DLINK: Dual link based radio frequency fingerprinting for wearable devices. In: Proceedings of IEEE Conference on Local Computer Networks (LCN). Clearwater Beach, FL, USA: IEEE; 2015. pp. 154-164

[8] Javali C, Revadigar G, Ding M, Jha S. Secret key generation by virtual link estimation. In: Proceedings of EAI International Conference on Body Area Networks (BodyNets). ICST (Institute for Computer Sciences, Social-Informatics and Telecommunications Engineering). Brussels, Belgium: ICST; 2015. pp. 63-72

[9] Bennett CH, Brassard G, Robert J-M. Privacy amplication by public discussion. SIAM Journal on Computing. 1988;**17**(2):210-229

[10] Ren Y, Chen Y, Chuah MC, Yang J. Smartphone based user verification leveraging gait recognition for mobile healthcare systems. In: Proceedings of Sensor, Mesh and Ad Hoc Communications and Networks (SECON). New Orleans, LA, USA: IEEE; 2013. pp. 149-157

Chapter 6

Using Smartphone Sensors for Localization in BAN

Julang Ying, Kaveh Pahlavan and Liyuan Xu

Additional information is available at the end of the chapter

http://dx.doi.org/10.5772/intechopen.80472

Abstract

Nowadays, various sensors are embedded in smartphone, making it a great candidate for localization applications. In this chapter, we explored and listed the localization sensors in smartphone, their characteristics, platforms, coordinate system and how they can be used in BAN. These sensors can be roughly divided into three types: physical IMU sensors (accelerometer, gyroscope and magnetometer), virtual IMU (gravity, step counter and electronic compass) and the environmental sensors (barometer, proximity and other miscellaneous). By applying different mathematical methods, the location of the target or the users can be calculated and used for further use, such as navigation, healthcare or military purpose.

Keywords: smartphone, sensors fusion, localization, BAN

1. Introduction

Nowadays, smartphones are open and programmable and come with a growing number of powerful embedded sensors, such as an accelerometer, digital compass, gyroscope, GPS, and camera, many of which, can be used for localization. In a typical BAN, the localization sensors measure certain characteristics related to the location of the phone to position it on a map [1]. These sensors either provide us information on the distance from reference points to help us calculate the absolute location, such as Received Signal Strength (RSS), Time-of-Arrival (TOA), Angle-of-Arrival (AOA) of RF signals or they provide us with the velocity and direction of movement from the motion sensors for calculation of displacement or the relative location of the object. One of the fundamental differences between the two methods is that the absolute localization needs an infrastructure of reference points but relative localization position the object relative to its previous location. **Figure 1** shows two examples of the results of localization using

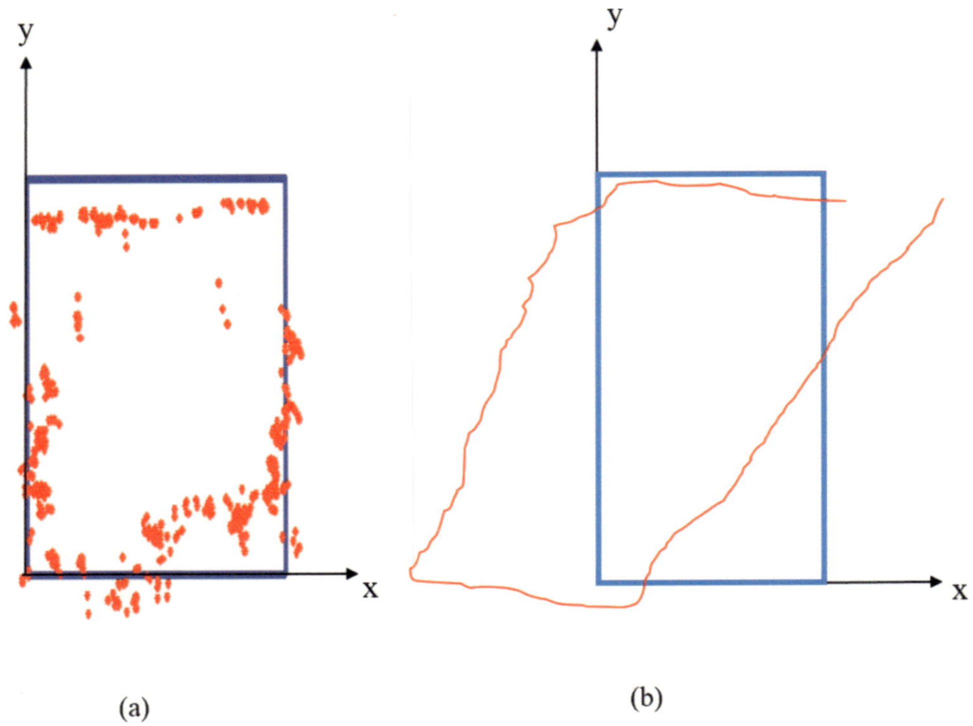

Figure 1. Results of localization with two classes of location sensing in square corridor route of an office (a) absolute localization using RSS of Wi-Fi access points (b) relative localization using IMU devices.

absolute and relative positioning systems [2] on a square route in a typical office building. **Figure 1b** shows the results of absolute Wi-Fi localization. The estimated locations (dots) are randomly distributed around the path of movement (solid line) of the object. **Figure 1b** shows the results of localization using an Inertia Motion Unit (IMU) device measuring the speed and direction of the movement. The estimated path of movement follow a straight line but, because of errors in angle and speed of movements, the location estimate gradually drifts from the actual path. Hybrid algorithms can combine the results of the two classes of sensors to achieve a more reliable navigation. These algorithms use the absolute localization to reduce the drift of IMU and use the IMU result to smooth the location estimates of the absolute location.

The most popular absolute positioning systems, such as Global Positioning System (GPS) and Wi-Fi Positioning System (WPS), sense features of the RF signals to measure the distance between the object and the reference points. The 26 satellites used as the reference points for GPS infrastructure are deployed for the purpose of positioning, while WPS opportunistically uses the Wi-Fi and cell phone signals for localization. Since absolute RF localization is the most fundamental and the most complex element of positioning, it is crucial to have a deep understanding of the behavior of RSS- and TOA-based ranging in different environments, which is well discussed in a great number of existing literature [3].

On the other hand, a typical application for relative positioning is Inertial Navigation Systems (INS). An INS uses a computer, motion sensors (accelerometers), rotation sensors (gyroscopes), and occasionally magnetic sensors (magnetometers) to continuously calculate by dead reckoning the position, the orientation, and the velocity (direction and speed of movement) of a moving object without the need for external references. With the development of technology, other methods can also be used for relative positioning. The speed of movement can be measured by number of rotations of the wheel (speedometer), Doppler spectrum of a received RF signal, the number of steps that a pedestrian walks (step counter), or similarities between the consecutive pictures taken by a camera.

Recently, Internet-of-Things (IOT) becomes a new fashion and opens up a new door to BAN localization. Large amount of IoT sensors have been deployed inside buildings, each of which has the ability to communicate and share location information to one other. Since the smartphone is able to communicate with both WiFi- and Bluetooth-based devices, its role in BAN localization becomes more and more important.

In this chapter, we present the way smartphone system visualize the location. We will also illustrate all the localization sensors in smartphone platform and discuss the characteristics of each. Examples are provided to show how these sensors are applied in the localization system and their accuracy is investigated as well.

2. Coordinate systems to visualize the location

In order to position a location on a map we need a coordinate system to visualize the location information. For global positing of a location, we need to refer to the global 3D coordinates of the earth. The most commonly 3D coordinates of the earth (**Figure 2**) are the geographical polar coordinates commonly referred to as: longitude, latitude and altitude (θ, ϕ, ρ). Longitude expresses angular deviation from east to west on the surface of the earth in degrees and latitude is the angular deviation from north to south in degrees. Elevation shows the distance from the center of the earth and it is usually given with respect of the sea level height. In the aerial vehicle applications elevation is referred to as altitude.

Ground navigation systems for outdoor and indoor areas track movements of the vehicles or robots on 2D maps such as layout of a floor of a building or 2D map of streets of an urban area in area for which altitude does not change substantially. Even in multi-floor 3D applications we use a 2D map with the floor number (a representative of altitude). Cartesian coordinates provide a better tool for visual tracking for most of popular applications in indoor and urban areas. Therefore, we usually convert longitude, latitude, and altitude to a Cartesian form using:

$$\begin{cases} X = \rho \times \cos(lat) \times \cos(lon) \\ Y = \rho \times \cos(lat) \times \sin(lon) \\ Z = \rho \times \sin(lat) \end{cases} \tag{1}$$

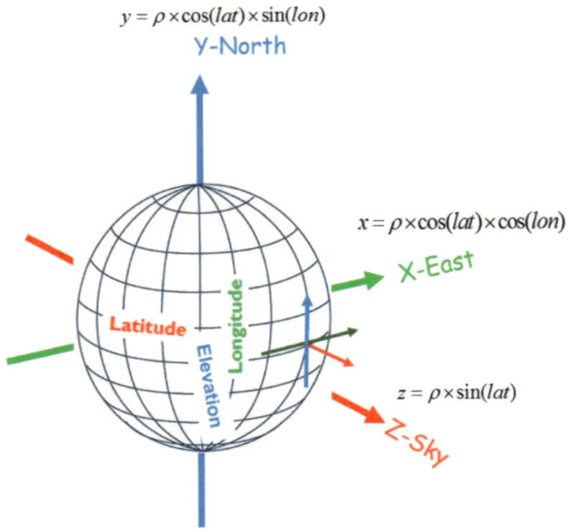

Figure 2. Earth 3D polar coordinate system with elevation, longitude and latitude.

In absolute positioning, a GPS or WPS location fix in polar or in Cartesian coordinate, represent a point in the 3D world frame coordinate. In relative positioning we represent the velocity and direction as vectors at each location. Accelerometers and gyroscopes are mechanical devices used for measurements of differential vectors for acceleration and rotation. We integrate the differential acceleration to determine the instantaneous velocity vector and we integrate the rotation vectors to determine the direction of motion.

In the universal Cartesian reference coordinate system, shown in **Figure 3a**, an acceleration or velocity vector in X-axis defines a vector tangential to the ground at the measurement sensor's current location pointing to the East. The vector in Y-axis is tangential to the ground at the measurement sensor's current location and pointing towards magnetic north. A vector in Z-axis points towards the sky and perpendicular to the ground at the location of the

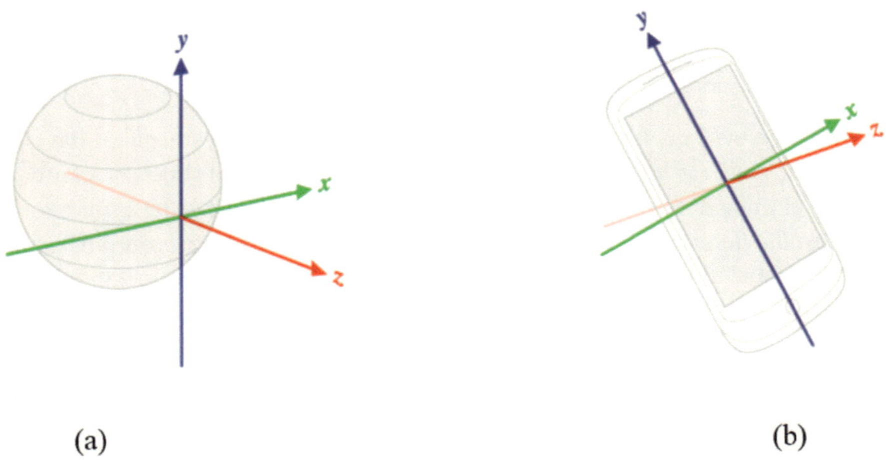

Figure 3. (a) Ground axis and (b) smartphone axis.

measurement sensor. However, as shown in **Figure 3b**, measurement sensors are MEM devices installed in a device, such as a smart phone, and their coordinates are defined relative to the device's screen and not the universal earth coordinate. When a device is held in its default orientation, the X-axis is horizontal and points to the right side of the device, the Y-axis is vertical and points up to the top of the device, and the Z-axis points towards the outside of the screen face. In this system, coordinates behind the screen have negative Z-values.

3. Sensors and platforms for opportunistic localization

Opportunistic localization is based on the location sensor payload of the platform we want to localize. Typical smart phones carry RF based GPS, Wi-Fi, Cell Phone, and iBeacon (Bluetooth Low Energy) chip sets, which support a variety of opportunistic RF localization capabilities for different environments and precision requirement. In addition, they carry a number of other sensors which can be used to enhance positioning of the device using traditional RF signals. **Table 1** shows typical sensors available in an Android device and their functionality if they are

Sensor name	Description	Type	Common uses
Barometer	Measures the atmospheric pressure in hPa (millibar)	Environment	Elevation for floor numbering
Ambient temperature	Measures ambient room temperature in degree Celsius	Environment	Detecting environment changes
Ambient light	Measures ambient light level in SI lux.	Environment	Detecting environment changes
Relative humidity	Measures relative ambient air humidity in percent	Environment	Detecting environment changes
Accelerometer	Measures the acceleration force in m/s^2 that is applied to a device on all three physical axes (x, y, and z), including the force of gravity	Mechanical	Motion detection (shake, tilt, etc.)
Gyroscope	Measures a device's rate of rotation in rad/s around each of the three physical axes (x, y, and z)	Mechanical	Rotation detection (spin, turn, etc.)
Step counters	Counts the number of steps taken by the person carrying the device	Mechanical	Measuring traveled distance
Magnetometer	Measures ambient geomagnetic field strength along the x,y,z axes in micro-Tesla (μT)	Electromagnetic	Creating a compass
Gravity	Measures the force of gravity in m/s^2 that is applied to a device on all three physical axes (x, y, z)	Electromagnetic	Motion detection (shake, tilt, etc.)
Proximity	Measures distance from the sensor to the closest visible surface measured in centimeters	Electromagnetic	Mapping the environment

Table 1. Typical sensors in an android smartphone.

used for localization. In addition to the traditional sensors such as gyroscope, magnetometer, accelerometer and barometer, there are sensors for ambient light, temperature, and humidity as well as force of gravity levels, proximity and step counts. The sensors can be beneficial for localization applications to enhance precision of RF localization. We can use the data collected by these sensors for 3D localization, calculation of speed and direction of movements and specifying the environment of operation. Positioning algorithms use RF location and motion information obtained from a variety of sensors. These sensors perform differently in different environments. For example, GPS which provides very reliable information for outdoor navigation does not operate deep in indoor areas. Therefore, in addition to the algorithm to determine the location, we need to have an algorithm to detect the environment to distinguish between the indoor and the outdoor environments. The data from all sensors is available as a resource to a positioning engineer to design different algorithms to achieve the precision requirements in the environment of operation.

The detailed description of these localization sensors is presented in the following sections as well as how accurate they can achieve in locating objects.

3.1. Accelerometer sensor

Accelerometer sensor measuring the acceleration (differential rate of variations of velocity) applied to a device in meter per square second (m/s^2) in the local Cartesian device coordinates (**Figure 3b**). **Figure 4a** shows the basic concept inside an accelerometer. A weight is hanging between two springs in a box and the displacement of the weight due to external forces moving the box is measured to calculate the acceleration in the direction of movement. The right side of **Figure 4c** shows how we can measure 3D acceleration of a plate carrying three accelerometer boxes placed in orthogonal directions.

Conceptually, an accelerometer measures the forces applied to the sensor in different directions and using Newton's second equation calculates the acceleration by dividing the force by mass of the sensor. When an IMU device rests in a place on a table in parallel to the earth surface, the

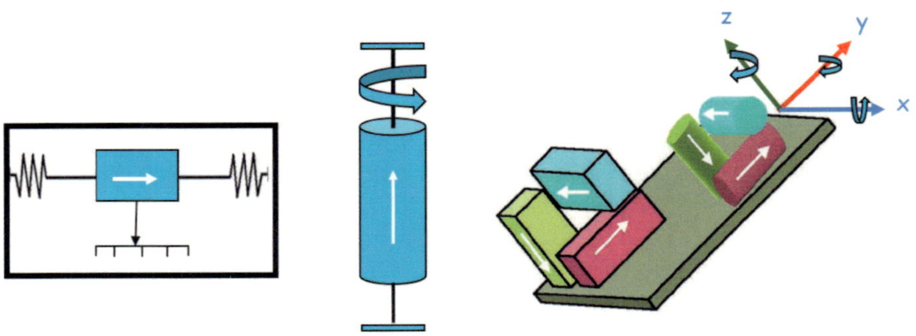

(a) (b) (c)

Figure 4. (a) Basic concept inside accelerometer (b) basic concept behind a gyroscope and (c) example of acceleration and rotation calculation.

accelerometer of the device should read a magnitude of $g = 9.81\ \mathrm{m/s^2}$, the gravity of the earth. When the IMU device is in free-fall and therefore accelerating towards the ground at $9.81\ \mathrm{m/s^2}$, its accelerometer should read a magnitude of $0\ \mathrm{m/s^2}$.

In order to measure the real acceleration of the device, also referred to as linear-acceleration, the contribution of the force of gravity must be eliminated. Applying a high-pass filter to the results of accelerometer readings eliminates the slow changes of the readings caused by gravity and detects the fast changes introduced by movements of the device. Conversely, using a low-pass filter isolates the force of gravity and eliminates the fast changes in the acceleration caused by the movements of the device.

3.2. Gyroscope sensor

Gyroscope sensor measure the differential rotation momentum around the local x, y, z axis of the device Cartesian coordinates in radians/second. **Figure 4b** shows the basic concept behind a gyroscope. A cylindrical mass is hanging around a central shaft like a wheel, as we change the direct wheel tits and we measure the angular displacement of the wheel. The coordinate system is the same as the one is used for the acceleration sensor. The right side of **Figure 4c** shows how we can measure the rotation in 3D around each of three axis of the device by placing three gyroscopes in orthogonal directions. The output of the gyroscope is integrated over time to calculate a rotation describing the change of angles over time.

Rotation is positive in the counter-clockwise direction. That is, an observer looking from some positive location on the x, y or z axis at a device positioned on the origin would report positive rotation if the device appeared to be rotating counter clockwise. If we refer to angular speed around the x-axis as ψ angular speed around the y-axis as θ and angular speed around the z-axis as ϕ (**Figure 5a**). The Euler transformation maps the accelerometer readings, $a(t)$, from the device coordinates to the universal coordinate:

$$\begin{bmatrix} a_X(t) \\ a_Y(t) \\ a_Z(t) \end{bmatrix} = \begin{bmatrix} \cos\theta\cos\psi & \sin\phi\sin\theta\cos\psi - \cos\phi\sin\psi & \cos\phi\sin\theta\cos\psi + \sin\phi\sin\psi \\ \cos\theta\sin\psi & \sin\phi\sin\theta\sin\psi + \cos\phi\cos\psi & \cos\phi\sin\theta\sin\psi - \sin\phi\cos\psi \\ -\sin\theta & \sin\phi\cos\theta & \cos\phi\cos\theta \end{bmatrix} \begin{bmatrix} a_x(t) \\ a_y(t) \\ a_z(t) \end{bmatrix} \quad (2)$$

Figure 5b shows a typical IMU device with both the device and the earth-fix coordinates. To find the location from the above equation we need to take a double integral. The first integration provides the velocity in each direction and the second integral provides the distance traveled by the device in each direction. Since smartphones are equipped with all the sensors mentioned above, we can consider them as a kind of smart IMU, and movement can be determined in the same way.

In practice, the gyroscope noise and offset will introduce some errors which need to be compensated for. This is usually done using the information from other sensors. The gyroscope cannot be emulated based on magnetometers and accelerometers, as this would cause it to have reduced local consistency and responsiveness. It must be based on a usual gyroscope

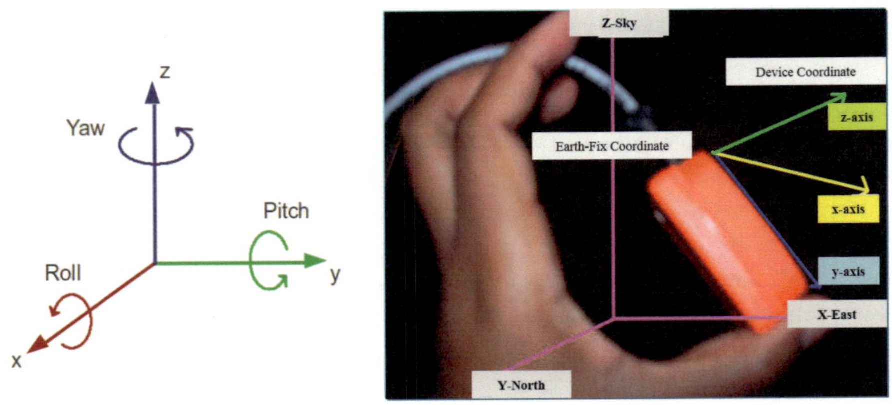

(a) (b)

Figure 5. (a) Definition of angular rotations: roll, pitch and yaw (b) a typical IMU device with local device coordinates.

chip. Most recent systems are of the strap down type, where the IMU sensor outputs are taken directly and processed to compute the orientation and displacement of the vehicle.

A simple laboratory experiment moving the IMU device shown in **Figure 6a** forward and then turning to the right. The IMU device is a relatively expensive device purchased in mid-2000 for approximately 3500 [4, 5]. **Figure 6b** and **c** shows the three dimensional readings of the gyroscope and accelerometer of the device. The gyroscope reads the pitch, yaw and roll in radian/second. The only rotation with this scenario of motion is around the z-axis for the yaw angle and pitch and roll remain at zero. Acceleration only has reading in x and y coordinates because we have no vertical motion. These values change ups and downs. **Figure 7a** and **b** shows the results first and second integral of the results after applying Euler's equation combining the results of accelerometer and the gyroscope (Eq. 2). The two figures represent the speed and traveled distance recorded by the laptop. The linear speed that is the square root of the sum of squares of the speeds on the x and y axes should remain relatively constant representing the speed of movement. **Figure 7c** shows the trajectory of the movement of the

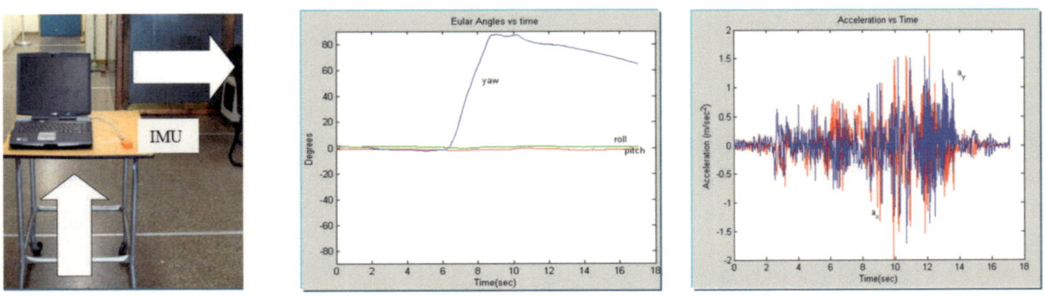

(a) (b) (c)

Figure 6. (a) Scenario of IMU movement, (b) readings of gyroscope angular movement and (c) readings of accelerometer.

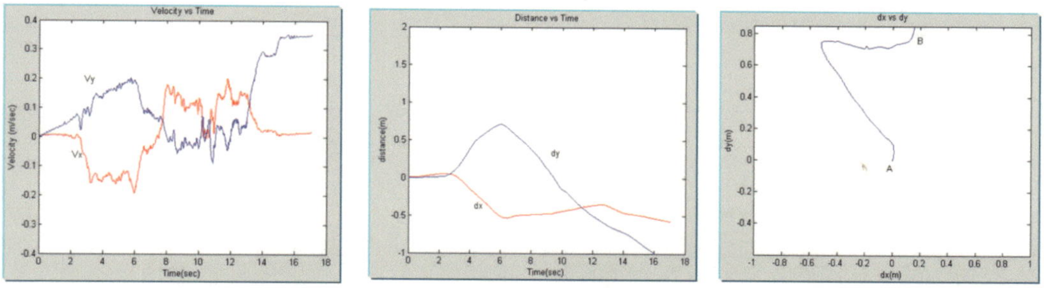

(a) (b) (c)

Figure 7. (a) Integral of the rotated movement (b) double integral representing motions in X and Y axis (c) trajectory of movement.

device as predicted from the results of IMU sensors readings. Results are similar to those of **Figure 1b**, which was obtained from another IMU unit.

3.3. Magnetometer

Magnetometer is a magnetic field sensor measuring the ambient magnetic field along the 3 sensor device local x, y and z axis in micro-Tesla (μT). Modern MEMS magnetometers measure the current induced in a coil due to changes in the magnetic field in the surrounding environment. **Figure 8a** shows the basic concept behind modern magnetometer devices. The intensity of the induced current in the coil is used as a measure for the strength of the magnetic field. **Figure 8b** shows how the 3D magnetic field can be measured with a device. Since magnetometers, measure strength and direction of magnetic field, they are also useful for measurement of the direction for localization and tracking. In the following sections we explain how we can design an electronic compass from readings of a MEMS magnetometer inside a smartphone.

3.4. Gravity sensor

Rather than high pass filtering, we low pass filter the measurements from an accelerometer we measure the force of gravity in the device coordinate. The magnitude of this vector is $9.81\ \mathrm{m/s^2}$ and its 3D (x, y, z) values reflect the effects of gravity on each of the three axis. These are values that we should subtract from the acceleration vector components to determine the linear acceleration. The value of the gravity vector in device coordinate is used for turning the smartphone and pads screens to be in parallel to the eye of the person reading the screen. Considering device coordinates shown in **Figure 3b**, if the gravity force along y-axis is the highest component, device is in up position and screen with smaller top is used. When the x-axis is the highest device is in the side position and the screen with long top is used. When device is resting on the floor z-axis is the largest value and the screen can be turned off. Results of gyroscope and magnetometer measurements are often used to complement the result of gravity force measurement obtained from the accelerometer. When the device is at rest, the output of the gravity sensor should be identical to that of the accelerometer.

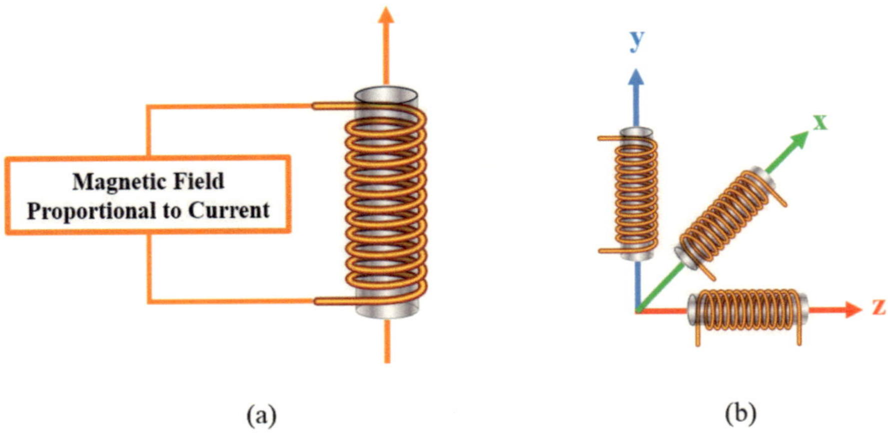

Figure 8. (a) Basic concept of a magnetometer and (b) implementation of a 3D magnetometer.

3.5. Step counter sensor

Step counter counts the number of steps taken by the pedestrian carrying a smart device such as a smartphone or a health monitoring band. The value is in integer and it reset to zero on a system reboot. The timestamp of the event is set to the time when the last step for that event was taken. The obvious application of this sensor is in fitness tracking applications but it is also useful for indoor geolocation using smart devices.

We can implement a step counter by using the measurements from an accelerometer. **Figure 9** shows hundred samples of magnitude of the accelerometer measurements for an Android phone. Considering Eq. 7.2, the magnitude of the acceleration is $a(t) = \sqrt{a_x(t)^2 + a_y(t)^2 + a_z(t)^2} - g$. **Figure 2a** shows the pattern of changes in acceleration between steps of a pedestrian carrying a device with accelerometer with hands. In each step first the pedestrian increase accretion of the body torso (carrying the hands and the device) using the landing foot and then she/he reduce the speed by applying negative acceleration to land on the other foot. As a result, variations of the magnitude of the accelerometer measurements follows a zigzag pattern on each step. We can detect the number of steps by counting the zigzags and that can be done either by peak detection or by detecting the zero crossing. With the peak detection algorithm we detect all peaks above a threshold and we select the highest in a window of time associated to the time for one step (**Figure 9a**). For zero crossing we find the intersect between the line representing the average acceleration and rising (or falling) parts of the plot (**Figure 9b**).

Using the step counter and the time stamps associated with each step, the average speed and the average step size can be determined and with that we can estimate the linear distance traveled by a pedestrian carrying a device with an accelerometer. To position the location of a pedestrian in a 2D map indoors or outdoors we also need to measure the rotations. Rotation can be measured with the results of gyroscope or the compass.

Figure 10 shows the results of an example relative localization system using the step counter and gyroscope of a typical smartphone at the third floor of the Atwater Kent Laboratory at the

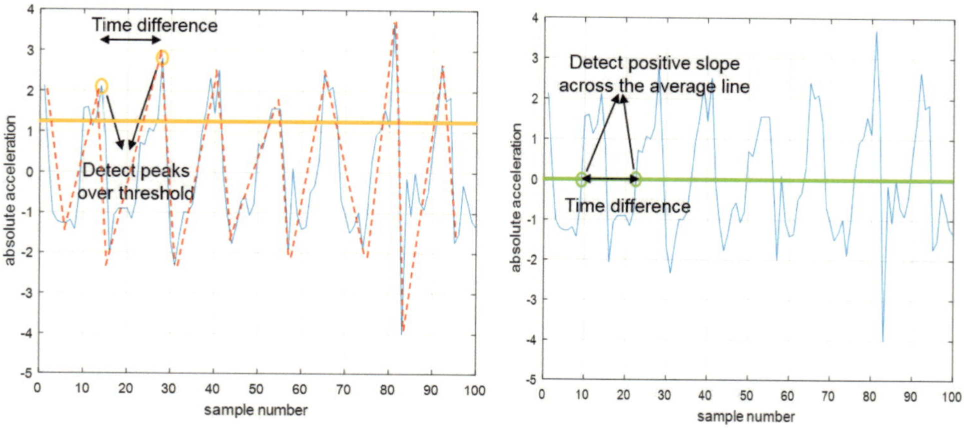

(a) (b)

Figure 9. (a) Step count using peak detection and (b) step count using zero crossing.

Worcester Polytechnic Institute. The schematic of corridors of this floor of building and layout of the exterior of the building in shown on the right figure. A user carrying the smartphone enters the floor from right to and walks straight and then around the central corridors before turning back to the original location. User holds the smartphone in front of the torso in parallel to the ground. In this posture the z-axis of the smartphone is towards the ceiling and the only rotation of the device is around this axis. **Figure 10a** shows the results of gyroscope readings in the three dimensions. There are four jumps in rotations around the z-axis (Azimuth or yaw) associated with four 900 turns in the route of movement of the device. The red line in **Figure 10b** illustrates the estimated path of movement when the results of step counts is complemented with the gyroscope readings. Typical increasing pattern of the drift of the location estimate away from the actual path of movement is observed. This type of error pattern is caused from using speed and direction of movement for relative localization and it is similar to the error pattern [6–8].

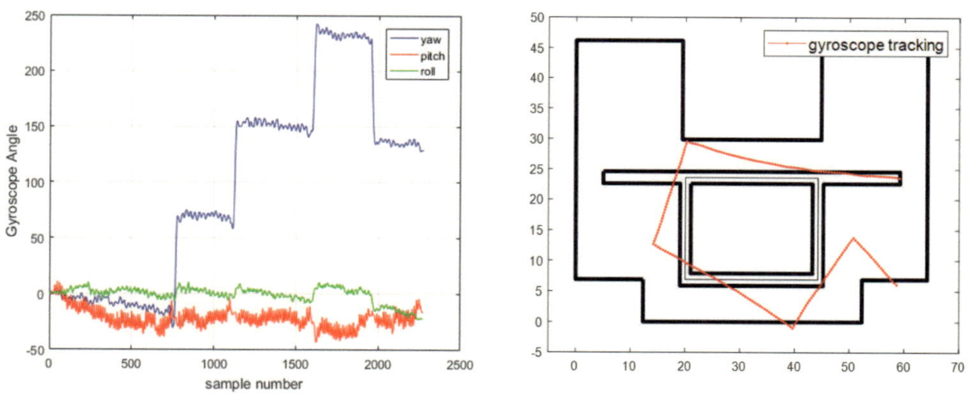

(a) (b)

Figure 10. (a) Results of a 3D gyroscope measurement and (b) localization using step count and gyroscope.

3.6. Electronic compass

Compass is one of the oldest mechanical magnetometer historically used for navigation. If we lay a compass in parallel to the earth surface the heading of the compass magnet points to the magnetic north. As a results, by rotating the compass to point towards a specific direction we measure the angle of that direction with respect to the magnetic north. This angle provides us with direction for relative navigation. A compass takes advantage of the earth electromagnetic field to determine the rotation angle of the device. Earth acts like a large dipole magnet with magnetic field lines originating from magnetic south pole (near the geographic south pole) and terminating in magnetic north pole located near the geographic north pole (**Figure 11a**). A compass has a small magnet in the center aligning with the magnetic north pole in all locations on the surface of the earth. The angle between the compass heading (the magnetic north) and the geographic north is called the magnetic declination angle (**Figure 11b**). The value of the decantation angle changes in location as well as in time. If we know the direction of geographical north in a location we can align the compass to that and measure the declination angle as the angle between the heading of the compass magnet and direction of the geometric north. In the east coast of United States inclination angle can go as low as $-22°$ (22°W) and on the west coast it can be as high as 22° (22.°E).

The National Oceanic and Atmospheric Administration (NOAA) has a public web calculator for calculation of magnetic declination angle around the Globe. Using this web site we read $-14°35'$W on December 22, 2017 in Newton, MA at a location with 130-ft elevation and longitude, latitude of (42°20′8″N, 71°12′14″W). Results indicate that the accuracy of values are within 22″ and the estimated value declines 4′E each year.

All popular smartphones in the market carry an electronically emulated compass application. These applications typically emulate the compass using the results of magnetometer, commonly available as a part of the IMU chip of the smartphone. **Figure 11a** shows a typical electronic compass implementation on an iPhone when the device is facing upward (z-axis of the device and the earth fix coordinates are aligned). The scaled round shape on top of the figure allows visualization of the angle between the north axis (y-axis) of the earth and the device to emulate the appearance of a compass. The Hx and Hy measurements of the magnetometer (**Figure 12b**) define the direction of compass heading in degrees using:

$$\theta = \begin{cases} 90 - \arctan\left(\dfrac{H_x}{H_y}\right) \times \dfrac{180}{\pi} & ; H_y > 0 \\ 270 - \arctan\left(\dfrac{H_x}{H_y}\right) \times \dfrac{180}{\pi} & ; H_y < 0 \\ 180° & ; H_y = 0, H_x < 0 \\ 0° & ; H_y = 0, H_x > 0 \end{cases} \tag{3}$$

As we turn the device around its z-axis, while laying the device on a table, the reading of the angle changes. For 346° ($-14°$) reading, shown in **Figure 12a**, the device heading points to the geographic north in Newton, MA which has a declination angle of approximately 14°.

http://dx.doi.org/10.5772/intechopen.80472

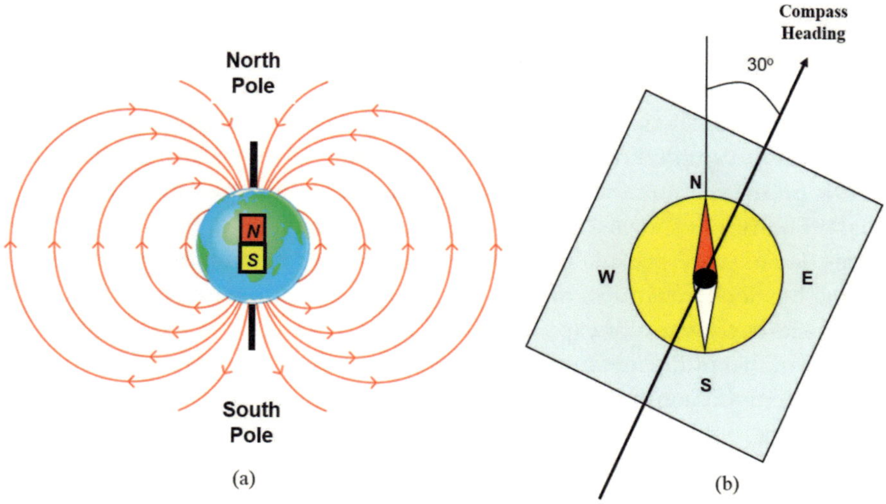

Figure 11. (a) Magnetic field of the Earth and North/South poles and (b) a traditional compass and heading angle.

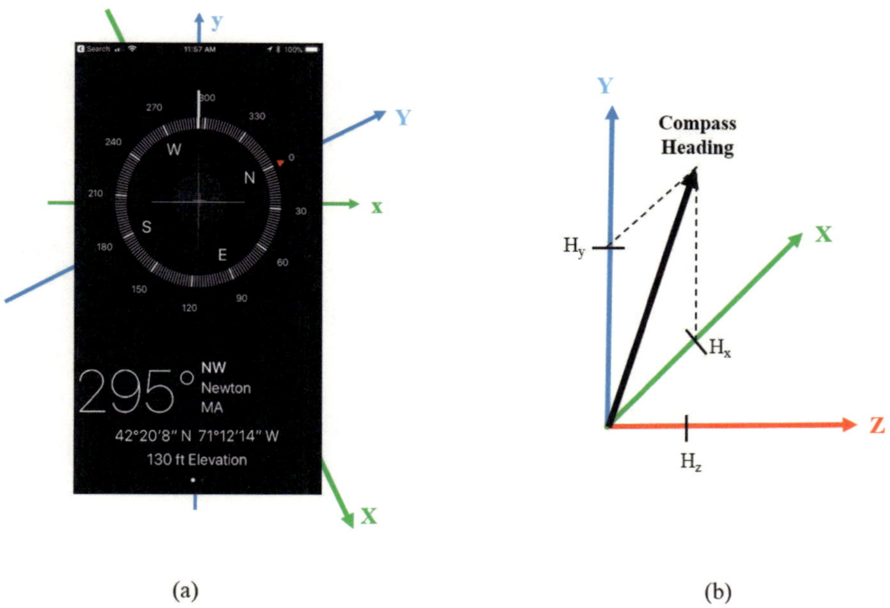

Figure 12. (a) Electronic compass application in smartphone and (b) compass heading and Earth coordinates.

3.7. Barometer

Barometer is a pressure sensor measuring the atmospheric pressure in hPa (millibar). Barometer is used to estimate elevation changes and consequently floor number of operation inside a multi-floor building. The relation between air pressure and height is given by [9]:

$$h \approx -\frac{R \times T_0}{g \times M} \times \ln\left(\frac{p}{p_0}\right) \tag{4}$$

Using Eq. (4) and parameters in **Table 2**, we can calculate altitude from air pressure. **Figure 13** shows the results of a smartphone barometer measurements in a typical 3-story office building. **Figure 13a** is produced from the results obtained in an elevator elevating three floors of the building and **Figure 13b** shows the results for climbing one floor of the building using stairs. Both figures demonstrate gradual change of the barometer reading during climbing up and down among the floors regardless of the speed and the pattern of motion. Range of variation of measurements in the elevator experiment for climbing three floors are approximately three times larger than that of the measurements for obtained from climbing one floor on the stairs. These observations demonstrate that barometer can be utilized to measure the change in altitude inside the buildings. **Figure 14** shows results of barometer measurements from a smartphone when a user carries the device in four floors of a typical office building in two different time of the same day. Pattern of measurement in different floors are clearly different allowing us to distinguish the floor of operation. However, results of barometer are corrupted by additive Gaussian noise, bias, and it is sensitive to the time of measurement [10, 11].

Parameter	Description	Value
p_0	Standard atmospheric pressure	101,325 Pa
R	Universal gas constant	8.31447 J/(mol·K)
T_0	Sea level standard temperature	288.15 K
g	Gravitation acceleration	9.81 m/s^2
M	Molar mass of dry air	0.0289644 kg/mol

Table 2. Parameters used for calculation of relation between height, h, and pressure, p.

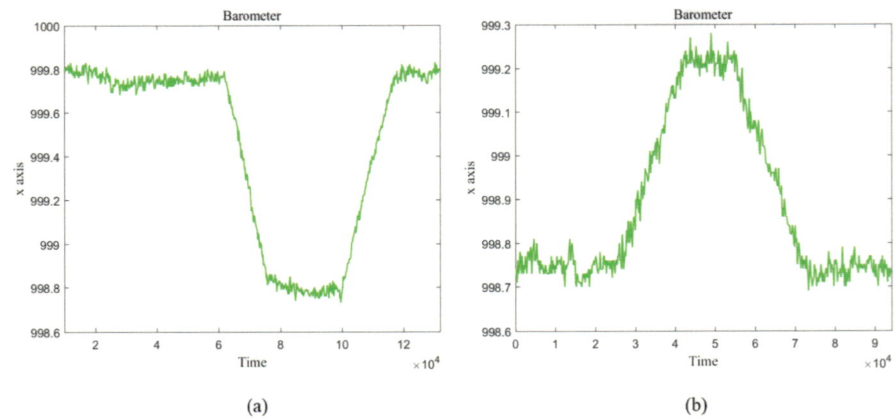

Figure 13. Barometric measurement in a typical 3-story building (a) elevating three floors of the building and (b) climbing floors using stairs.

http://dx.doi.org/10.5772/intechopen.80472

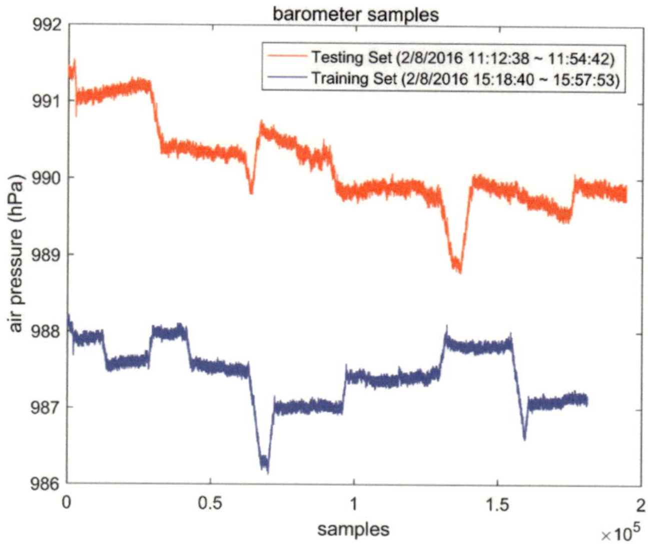

Figure 14. Barometric reading at different time.

Methods to mitigate these effects and have a better estimate of the floor number in an office building is discussed in [9].

Author details

Julang Ying[1]*, Kaveh Pahlavan[1] and Liyuan Xu[2]

*Address all correspondence to: jying@wpi.edu

1 Worcester Polytechnic Institute, Worcester, USA

2 University of Science and Technology, Beijing, China

References

[1] Pahlavan K, Li X, Makela J-P. Indoor geolocation science and technology. IEEE Communications Magazine. 2002;**40**(2):112-118

[2] He J, Geng Y, Pahlavan K. Toward accurate human tracking: Modeling time-of-arrival for wireless wearable sensors in multipath environment. IEEE Sensors Journal. 2014;**14**(11): 3996-4006

[3] He J, Geng Y, Liu F, et al. CC-KF: Enhanced TOA performance in multipath and NLOS indoor extreme environment. IEEE Sensors Journal. 2014;**14**(11):3766-3774

[4] Iadanza E, Dori F, Miniati R, et al. Patients tracking and identifying inside hospital: A multilayer method to plan an RFId solution. In: 30th Annual International Conference of the IEEE Engineering in Medicine and Biology Society (EMBS). IEEE; 2008. pp. 1462-1465

[5] Liu G, Geng Y, Pahlavan K. Effects of calibration RFID tags on performance of inertial navigation in indoor environment. In: International Conference on Computing, Networking and Communications (ICNC). IEEE; 2015. pp. 945-949

[6] Pahlavan K, Krishnamurthy P, Geng Y. Localization challenges for the emergence of the smart world. IEEE Access. 2015;**3**:3058-3067

[7] Alemdar H, Ersoy C. Wireless sensor networks for healthcare: A survey. Computer Networks. 2010;**54**(15):2688-2710

[8] Wang Y, Fu R, Ye Y, et al. Performance bounds for RF positioning of endoscopy camera capsules. In: IEEE Topical Conference on Biomedical Wireless Technologies, Networks, and Sensing Systems (BioWireleSS). IEEE; 2011. pp. 71-74

[9] Ying J, Ren C, Pahlavan K. On automated map selection problem in indoor navigation for smart devices. In: Proceedings of the IEEE Telecommunications Summit; 2015

[10] Pahlavan K, Levesque AH. Wireless Information Networks. John Wiley & Sons; 2005

[11] Geng Y, Pahlavan K. Design, implementation, and fundamental limits of image and RF based wireless capsule endoscopy hybrid localization. IEEE Transactions on Mobile Computing. 2016;**15**(8):1951-1964

Chapter 7

Systems of Preventive Cardiological Monitoring: Models, Algorithms, First Results, and Perspectives

Sergey Kirillov, Aleksandr Kirillov, Vitalii Iakimkin, Michael Pecht and Yuri Kaganovich

Additional information is available at the end of the chapter

http://dx.doi.org/10.5772/intechopen.75921

Abstract

The results of work on creating methods, models, and computational algorithms for remote preventive health-monitoring systems are presented, in particular, cardiac preventive monitoring. The main attention is paid to the models and computational algorithms of preventive monitoring, the interaction of the computing kernels of a remote cluster with portable ECG recorders, implantable devices, and sensors. Computational kernels of preventive monitoring are a set of several thousand interacting automata of analog of Turing machines, recognizing the characteristic features and evolution of the hidden predictors of atrial fibrillation(AF), ventricular tachycardia or fibrillation (VT-VF), sudden cardiac death, and heart failure (HF) revealed by them. The estimation of the time for reaching the heart events boundaries is calculated on the basis of the evolution equations for the ECG multi-trajectories determined by recognizing automata. Evaluation time of heart event (HE) boundaries to achieve is calculated on the basis of the evolution equations for ECG multi-paths defined by recognizing machines. Ultimately, the computational cores reconstruct the ECG of the forecast and give temporary estimates of its achievement. Cloud computing cluster supports low-cost ECG ultra-portable recorders and does not limit the possibilities of using a more complex patient telemetry containing wearable and implantable devices: CRT and ICD, CardioMEMS HF System, and so on.

Keywords: preventive monitoring, heart failure prognosis, remote calculating cluster, optimize drug therapy

1. Introduction

The growing interest in remote cardiac-monitoring systems is associated primarily with the need for an early prognosis in the development of heart failure (HF) disease [1] and an early prognosis of developing against the background HF of such heart events as atrial fibrillation (AF), ventricular tachycardia or fibrillation (VT-VF), and sudden cardiac death [2]. In addition, on the assumption that remote monitoring systems can effectively cope with prognostic tasks, the next call to remote monitoring systems occurs namely the development and optimization of risk reduction strategies and the strategy of drug or device cardioversions. It is about the management of the patient's cardiac condition through a drug or a device therapy, determining the degree of effectiveness of therapy and predicting the results of treatment [3]. However, despite the significant advances and new promising results [4] in the field of management and effective prevention, there are a significant number of problems associated with the lack of a physiologically justified mathematical model of management. There is some analog of the problems described earlier in the problems of engineering asset management (EAM). The basis of EAM is Prognostics and Health Management (PHM) systems, including also algorithms of predictive analytics, big data, deep learning, and so on. Another component of EAM is represented by Intelligent Maintenance Systems (IMS); here the main goal is to develop systems of preventive maintenance, self-maintenance, and self-recovery systems. Technical systems are somewhat simpler than biomechanical systems, so the mathematical PHM models, developed for the prognosis, are more formalized, including in the field of physics of failure. A simple mechanical transfer of PHM models is hardly possible, but some useful analogies are appropriate. In particular, in setting the tasks of calculating optimizing strategies for preventive maintenance, estimating the time to reach the boundaries of the mechanisms dysfunction and the failure boundary, and so on. In this chapter, some useful formulations and models of the PHM will be used as applied. The noted analogy can be supplemented by fact that used in cardioversion the devices are both wearable and implanted also need a prognosis of their failures and dysfunctions. As a result, the complex task of constructing PHM models for the system "biomechanical object plus implantable device or sensor" is relevant for the further development of preventive cardiac-monitoring systems.

Finally, the goal of PCM applications in medicine, using mHealth and eHealth platforms with telemetry transfer capabilities to a remote server and a large computational resource in the form of distributed computing systems, the cloud computing service, is reduced to the following:

1. based on the chronological database of each patient and current data, to calculate the parameters or predictors that characterize the evolution of HF;
2. on the same database, predict the appearance of hidden HF predictors (i.e., the appearance and evolution of those ECG signal characteristics that precede the appearance of HF);
3. to reveal the hidden predictors of cardiac events, namely AF, VT-VF, and sudden cardiac death;
4. to determine evolutionary equations for hidden predictors and estimate the time to reach the predicted characteristics of the ECG.

Similarly, remote systems of preventive monitoring should be aimed at solving management tasks, that is, constructing a strategy for variable parameters with drug therapy or programming CRT, IDC devices.

If to consider the problems noted earlier in the context of preventive monitoring, then the question of developing the systems of preventive maintenance strategies must be raised.

Thus, the prognosis of heart conditions is now reduced to the identification of predictors (ECG characteristics) cardiac events, which, in fact, have to answer the question of how likely the presence and numerical characteristics of ECG predictors provide the appearance of cardiac events. Such predictors include the length of the CT of the interval, the CT dispersion, the P-wave index, and so on. A new trend, known as nonlinear dynamics methods, adds to the existing predictors of the entropy characteristics commonly used in nonlinear dynamics for the classification of trajectories of dynamic systems. These include fractal, dimensional, and entropy characteristics, for example, information dimension, approximation entropy, and so on. The methods of symbolic dynamics are also used, the essence of which is reduced to the study of dynamical systems on the basis of the analysis of symbolic cascades. There are some results in the cases where the cascade is a topological Markov chain. At the same time, transferring results from cascades to a dynamic system requires that the dynamic symbolic system is the factor system.

In addition, there is no model of cardiac activity tied to a specific system of dynamic equations. Ultimately, the prediction achieved by measuring or calculating the predictors mentioned requires a number of conditional transitions, that is, the fulfillment of a multitude of conditions involving various facts from an anamnesis, the general state of the organism, the presence or absence of a range of diseases, which reduces the effectiveness of the prediction up to the phrase "positive prognosis" and "negative prognosis.".

Section 1 briefly describes the basic model of the propagation of the action potential (AP). The presented equation for the AP is purely a model, more realistic models; for example, Microdomain model [5] is not considered since the main purpose of this section is to demonstrate the result of numerical simulation of the propagation of AP on the basis of bundle cellular automata. Equations for ion currents are placed in the bundle of automata, which makes it possible to locally vary the parameters of the ion current models, the degree of anisotropy, and the local geometry of the cardio tissue [6]. In the context of this chapter, this section allows to refer to the microscopic theory of ion currents and action potential, without which the formal operation with this series of ECG wavelet coefficients is enriched by an innumerable number of possible scenarios for constructing recognizing automata.

Section 2 describes the evolution of wavelet coefficients in models of random walking on a multidimensional lattice and on a multidimensional continuum. With some realistic assumptions, it is possible to estimate the time to reach the boundaries of cardiac events or HF. The transition to high dimensions is also due to attempts of detection predictors of trajectories for the prognosis of rotors in AF.

Approximation entropy is given considerable attention in [7]. However, approximation entropy in principle is conceived as some estimate of Kolmogorov complexity. Moreover, K-complexity is an algorithmically unsolvable quantity, which encourages researchers to seek estimates for K-complexity in the form of various kinds of entropies, for example, Shannon entropy.

It should be noted that in reality, an estimate of not K-complexity but of conditional K-complexity is required, which induces the transitions from the time series of wavelet coefficients to vector processes.

There are other good reasons to go to the vector process in connection with the prognostic tasks and estimation of the time to reach. The automatic transfer of the random walk theory over multidimensional lattices and the multidimensional continuum [8, 9] is hampered by the fact that these models were created for problems in the theory of polymers, where the length of the jump is constant and equal to the length of the monomer. The situation is partly saved by the introduction of the distribution function of jumps along the lengths. For the visibility of finite formulas, it was necessary to introduce the averaged length of the jump. However, the main goal of this section is to construct multidimensional state spaces and then sets of trajectories on them. In such spaces of HF regions, the cardiac events are clearly distinguished by wavelet coefficient values. However, the Euclidean metric is not quite suitable for estimating the closeness of trajectories. Therefore, in Section 2, we give an example of the bifurcations of the distribution of density function on the basis of the elementary catastrophe theory.

Section 3 describes the construction of family of recognition automata and gives an example of an evolution equation for the internal states of automata. Here, the models described in Sections. 1 and 2 contribute to the understanding and further formalization of the principles of constructing recognizing automata and their operation. Since in algorithmic realizations of automata, only principles are laid down. All their further activities including reproduction, an increase in complexity, self-learning, and adaptation (in the context of personalized cardiology) should occur as a result of self-organization based on the principles laid down in the algorithms.

Section 5 describes the interaction of recognizing automata with peripheral devices, wearable or implanted, and also possibly other body sensors. It shows how the transmission and processing of ECG signals occurs and as a family of automata forms signaling automata and places them on portable devices. In turn, the automata, delivered to the device, control the calculations on a remote family of automata.

Section 6 is devoted to verification and discussion of the results and conditions for a correct prognosis.

Section 7 is devoted to the formalization of trajectories management tasks. The management model is outlined in the language of homotopy theory and the theory of infinite loop spaces. It considers the set of all admissible trajectories and the possibility of continuous deformation of some trajectories into others, as well as possible obstacles to such deformation. It is intuitively clear that the singularities that arouse in the model must be associated with the birth of filaments in models AF-VT. However, this fact is not rigorously proved in this chapter. Hope is encouraged by the fact that filaments, like singularities in the base space, are of a homotopic nature in both cases and, therefore, are invariant with respect to any deformations, which means that they can be recorded by ECG analysis on the body.

The traditional approach to the diagnosis and prognosis of heart event (HE) based on an ECG can be found in [10, 11] and references cited therein. Summarizing the goal of PHM applications in preventive cardiac monitoring is reduced not only to accurate estimates of the time to reach the boundaries of cardiac events. One of PHM tasks is managing the state of complex systems and determining optimal management strategies to extend the lifetime of complex technical objects. Consequently, in the PHM cardiac applications, the PHM task is also the creation of models and management algorithms, that is, the retention of multitrajectories of cardiac states in classes of trajectories without cardiac events. How much such task is possible is discussed in the last section of this chapter in the framework of the topological model of trajectory management.

2. Basis

The construction of automata recognizing hidden, early predictors of cardiac events is determined by a set of requirements that follow from the basic models and representations. The basic principles should include the basic models describing the propagation of the action potential in cardio tissue [12, 13] and the models of ionic membrane currents [14]. Formula (1) represents a simplified equation for the action potential

$$\frac{\partial V(r,t)}{\partial t} = -D\Delta V(r,t) + I_{ion}(r) \tag{1}$$

V is the transmembrane potential, D is the homogeneous pseudo-diffusion constant of the intracellular gap junctional coupling, I_{ion} (r) is the total transmembrane ionic current, and Δ is the Laplace operator.

There are also more general models that take into account inhomogeneous cellular structure, mentioned in Section "Introduction."

Using the models of ion transport through biological membranes based on models of statistical thermodynamics of nonequilibrium processes [13], a digital model of bundle cellular automata is created. The bundle cellular automata in their continuum limit represent a smooth fiber bundle [15]. In this case, the diffusion part of the "reaction–diffusion" equation is determined in the base manifold of the bundle. In the fibers, the anisotropic architecture of myocardial regions was modeled. Different fibers of bundle cellular automata corresponded to different degrees of anisotropy and different geometric configurations. The results of numerical simulation are shown in **Figure 1**.

The main result obtained by numerical simulation is reduced to demonstrating the growth of wavefront fluctuations and fluctuations in the curvature of the wavefront after repeated passage of the front along the same macroscopic myocardial regions, that is, the model of bundle cellular automata, and in the continuum limit of smooth fiber bundle is an acceptable approximation in the problem of macroscopic description of the evolution of the wavefront of the AP, taking into account the changes taking place on the cellular, microscopic scale, when changing the microgeometry of cell bonds and the variation in the parameters of the microscopic model of intercellular conductivity by multiplicative noise, as was done in the work [16] in the model of Khodzhin-Huxley axon with Markov dichotomous voltage noise.

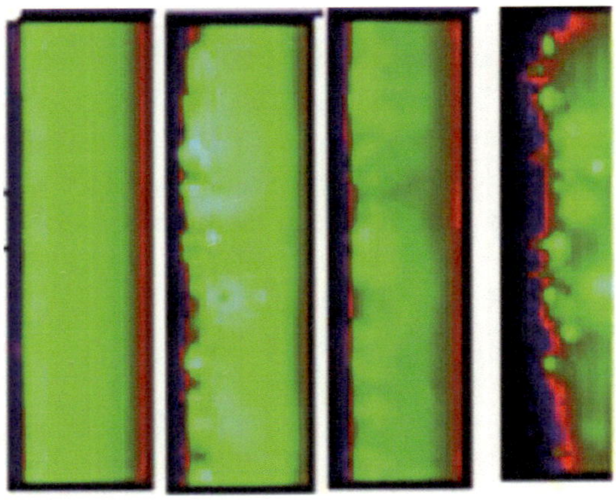

Figure 1. The results of numerical simulation.

Models of the AP by individual cells and its conduction from cell to cell through intercellular gap junctions are discussed in the work in [12].

3. Model

Another basis for constructing prediction algorithms and recognizing automata is the random walk model on a multidimensional lattice or in a multidimensional continuum. Thus, at each set of R-R intervals of a fixed ECG length, the signal is represented as a set of its wavelet coefficients

$$\left\{ {}^{k}_{Hist}W^{N}_{i,j} \right\}, N = 1, 2, 3, \ldots, N^{*} \quad (2)$$

N is the number of R-R cycle, i, j are indexes of wavelet decomposition, *Hist* is the heart rate histogram column index, and k is the numbering of vectors from wavelet coefficients of dimension N^*.

Moreover, for all fixed indices except N, stochastic process with discrete time, N cascade, is determined. Further, fixing the limiting value N as N^* is determined by a set of vectors of dimension N^*, chosen from the consistent values of the process under consideration with discrete time. As a result, the space $\boldsymbol{R}^{N^*}$ is determined, consisting of all possible finite segments of dimension размерности N^*

$$\{\boldsymbol{R}_k\} \overset{\text{def}}{=} \left\{ {}^{\text{k}}_{\text{Hist}}W^{N:\ kN^* \le N \le (k+1)N^*, k=0,1,2,3\ldots}_{i,j} \right\}, \ \boldsymbol{R}_k \in \boldsymbol{R}^{N^*} \quad (3)$$

The total number of such spaces $\boldsymbol{R}^{N^*}$ corresponds to the product of the number of elements of sets $\{Hist\}$, $\{i\}$, $\{j\}$.

Thus, the formed product of spaces contains the set of all admissible values of any ECG signals (set of admissible states). In this set, there is a subset containing sequences of cardiac events (CE) и HF predictors. Such a subset is formed by wavelet coefficients from the ECG database of cardiac events и HF predictors. Thus, each finite segment of any process is typed by elementary transitions in each coordinate $\boldsymbol{R}_k \in \boldsymbol{R}^{N^*}$, if the probability of such transition is known. For the transition, one vector of dimension N^* to another is required, N^* transitions. As a result, the initial vector goes into another vector. If the probabilities of elementary transitions are known, the probability from vector to vector is determined by the product of elementary coordinate-wise probabilities. Successive transitions from one vector to another form of the trajectory in space of the product. In each product space, the probability density of the transition is determined, expressed as a Feynman path integral. A vector in each fixed product space is defined as a state, and a sequence of vectors determines the state trajectory. The set of states in the product of spaces defines a multistate, a multitrajectory, respectively.

The introduction of the probability density of transition from one state to another is interpreted as a random walk of a trajectory in state spaces. Thus, the problem of predicting cardiac events is reduced to the calculation of the probability of transition to the boundary of the region obtained by mapping the ECG from the base of cardiac events into a product of spaces. In addition to a subset of cardiac events clearly expressed by their ECG (AF-VF) in the space of events, regions corresponding to various changes in the point-wise Holder regularity are also separated relatively to the regularity characteristics for the ECG norm. The procedure of allocation of such regions is performed during the monitoring and based on two microlocal spaces [17]. Therefore, the prognosis is reduced to calculating the probability density function (PDF) for transition probabilities from one state to another ($\boldsymbol{R}_k \rightarrow \boldsymbol{R}_{k+1}$). Since the regions of cardiac events and the irregular behavior of the ECG signal are separated, the probability of transition of the state to the boundary of the "critical" regions in L (L is the continuous analog of the number of cardiac cycles) steps is calculated. At the difficulty of calculating the probability density function, calculations are carried out for the moments of the PDF or the cumulants. The time required to reach the "critical region" is determined from explicit analytical expressions for the second moment of PDF.

Evolutionary equations for the probability density are derived from the Feynman representation of the PDF under certain limiting assumptions, in particular, the Fokker-Planck equation, and the equations for single-step processes. The calculation of the Feynman integral also reduces to solutions of the Hamilton-Jacobi equation, the Schrödinger equation, and the WKB method [18].

However, in the multidimensional case, the solution of the equations is possible only numerically and generates some computational problems.

In [19], on the basis of modification of random walk models [8, 9], the PDF of transition probabilities (probability function of end-to-end distribution) представлено as the Feynman path integral

$$P(\boldsymbol{R}_0, \boldsymbol{R}_L, L) = \int_{\boldsymbol{r}(0)=\boldsymbol{R}_0}^{\boldsymbol{r}(L)=\boldsymbol{R}_L} \mathcal{D}[\boldsymbol{r}(s)] \exp\left[-\int_0^L ds \langle \xi \rangle_L \boldsymbol{r}_L^2(s)\right] \tag{4}$$

$\boldsymbol{r}_L(s)$ is the parameterization of polygonal $\{\Delta \boldsymbol{R}_i; \mathrm{i} = 1, 2, 3 \ldots\}$ and L is the continuous analog of the number of cardiac cycles.

On the basis of such representations, second moments of the PDF are analytically calculated, which allows to determine the average time to reach the HE boundaries, represented by formulas (6)–(8). Presented cases of analytical expressions take into account not all possible scenarios for the evolution of states, in particular, the fact of the appearance of obstacles to the realization of certain types of trajectories, as a result of degradation of the cardio tissue, is not taken into account.

To solve these problems, we introduce a one-step cascade operator, defined as follows:

$(\boldsymbol{r}_1, \ldots \boldsymbol{r}_m, \ldots \boldsymbol{r}_{N^*}, \boldsymbol{r}_{N^*+1}, \ldots)$ - cascade

$$\Omega^* \left(..m_i..\right) = m_i + 1 \tag{5}$$

$$\left(\Omega^*\right)^{N^*} \boldsymbol{R}_k = \boldsymbol{R}_{k+1}, \forall k$$

The introduced operator has an analog in the symbolic space on the basis of which the recognizing automata, which is presented in the next section, are constructed.

Within the framework of the presented model of the segment wander from the wavelet coefficients of the ECG signal and in the performance of the Markov property, the prediction and estimates of the time to reach the boundaries of the regions of dysfunctions or cardiac events of AF-HF type are obtained by inferring the probability density from the Feyman representation. In some cases, the Fokker-Planck equations are obtained. By solving these equations, or by calculating the end-to-end distribution function by the methods described in the paper [8, 9], the following estimates of the time to reach the boundaries (L_{time}) events are obtained:

1. Models of the free random walk.

$$L_{time} = \frac{< \|\boldsymbol{R}^C\|^2 >^2}{(N^* - 1)\langle \xi \rangle}, \tag{6}$$

1. Models of random walk with constraints. Under condition of confirmation of hypothesis of model of random walk with constraints, the estimation of L_{time} is determined as a solution of equation

$$< \|\boldsymbol{R}^c\|^2 >= 2\left\{\Theta L_{time} - \Theta^2\left[1 - e^{-L_{time}/\Theta}\right]\right\}, \Theta = \frac{const}{\langle \xi \rangle (N^* - 1)} \tag{7}$$

1. Models of random walk in a non-simply-connected domain. Under condition of confirmation of a hypothesis of model of random walk in a non-simply-connected domain, estimates of L_{time} is determined as a solution of equation

$$< \|\boldsymbol{R}^c\|^2 >= \langle \xi \rangle^{1/(N^*+2)} \left(\frac{N^* + 2}{3} \sqrt{\frac{2\langle \xi \rangle}{N^*}} L_{time}\right)^{6/N^*+2} \tag{8}$$

where $\boldsymbol{R}^C \in \{border\ of\ HE, HF\}$, $< \|\boldsymbol{R}^c\|^2 >$ 2-th moment probability function of end-to-end distribution; $\langle \xi \rangle$is the average length of an elementary transition.

Similar to the previous ones, it is advisable to construct the space of events and the symbolic space for a continuous analog of the wavelet transform. The transition to the continual version requires much computing power, but it has some advantages. **Figure 2** shows the value of the wavelet coefficients of the continuous wavelet transformation. Only in this case is the development successful of the multiscale fluctuations of the QRS complex by the scaling variable in a patient with persistent AF. The prognosis of the development of such fluctuations and the time to reach the value by the wavelet coefficients of fields of strong irregularity according to Hölder are also modeled in terms of a random walk on a multidimensional lattice or in a continuum.

Let us return to the one-dimensional processes of wavelet coefficients with a fixed quadruple of indices. The PDF of these processes determines the probability of an elementary jump under the action of the shift operator by one step, that is, eventually the probability of a transition for L steps, as in the case of the vector process considered earlier. The type of distribution density thus affects the construction of the trajectory of the vector process. Here, it is necessary to note the following: in those cases when the one-dimensional process under consideration is a Markov diffusion process, and on the part of the wavelet coefficients of the ECG signal it is. The distribution density function here is a stationary solution of the Fokker-Planck equation. Also assume, for example, that the stationary solution is expressed as an exponential function of some potential function [16].

$$P_s(x) = const\cdot\exp\left(U(x)\right) \tag{9}$$

where x is some wavelet cascade in a continuum limit.

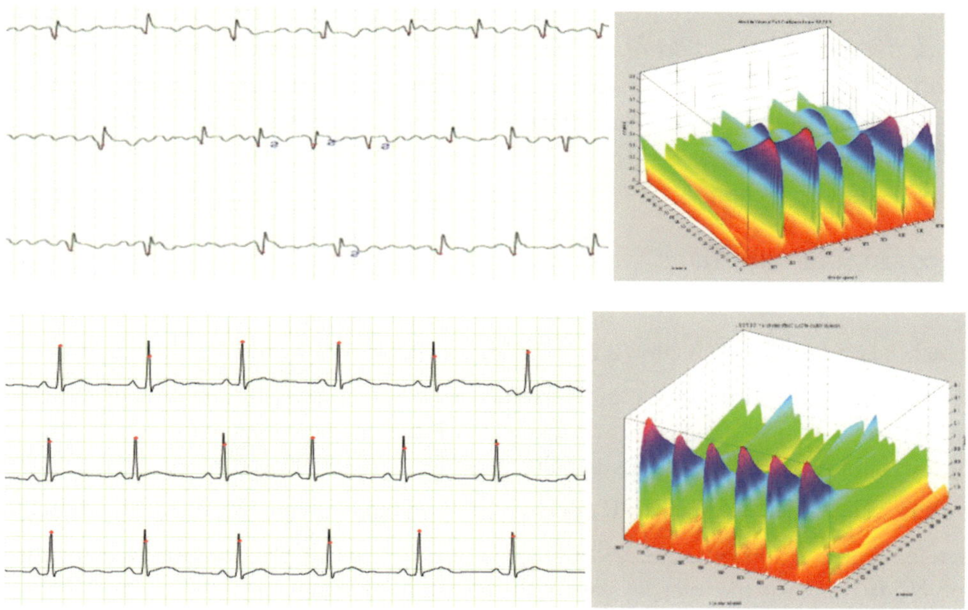

Figure 2. Continuous wavelet transformation of ECG with AF and ethalon.

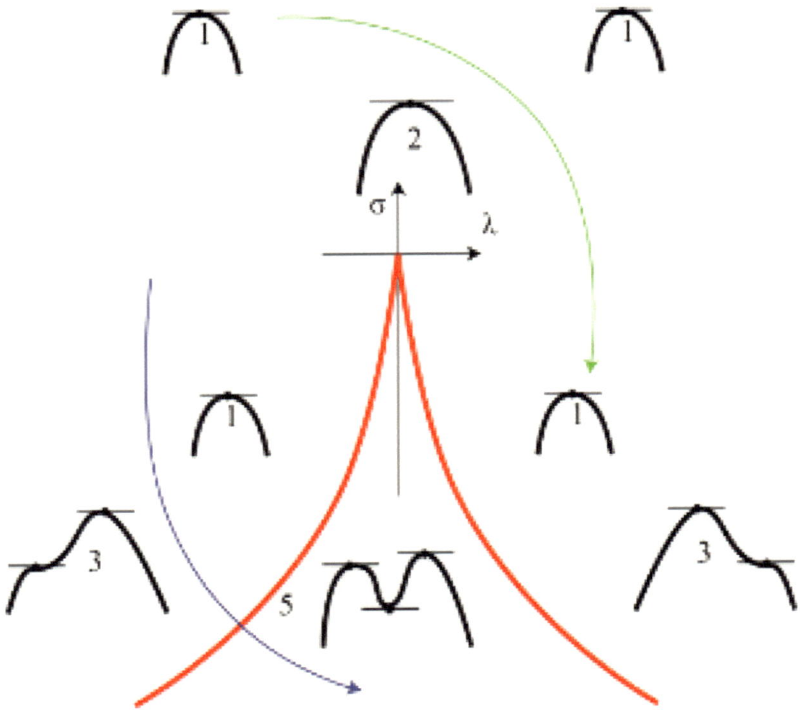

Figure 3. The sets of bifurcations or catastrophes and the changing of type of the PDF.

In this case, it is possible to calculate possible rapid transformations of the PDF of one type, another type using elementary constructions from the theory of catastrophes (Poston Stewart) For this, the potential function or the neighborhood of its maximum is approximated by a polynomial of the fourth order. As a result of standard transformations (Poston), the so-called bifurcation set on the plane of the approximating polynomial coefficients is constructed, as shown in **Figure 3**.

4. Recognizing automata

For each cascade $\left\{ {}^{k}_{Hist}W^{N}_{i,j} \right\}, N = 1, 2, 3, \ldots, N^*$, an additional symbolic affine space S^{n+1} is defined, the dimension of which is determined as $n + 1$ number of columns of the cascade histogram, that is, each histogram of the wavelet coefficient values with a fixed triplet of indices (*Hist, i, j*) is a point in the symbolic space S^n. This point determines the internal state of the automata. An elementary shift operator, shifting the segment $\left\{ {}^{k}_{Hist}W^{N}_{i,j} \right\}, N = 1, 2, 3, \ldots, \infty$ by one in the direction of index N^* growth, is also defined at preservation of a segment of length N^*. In this case, the internal state of the automata changes, the point in space shifts. The state of the automata changes with an elementary shift by the transition of elementary value from one coordinate to another, that is, in the case of a shift, the transition of elementary value from one column of the histogram to another column is carried out. By construction, the elementary transition is equivalent to the shift operator of some initial segment in segment $\left\{ {}^{k}_{Hist}W^{N}_{i,j} \right\}, N = 1, 2, 3, \dots, \infty$ by a unit step. In a symbolic space, the elementary shift corresponds to the multiplication of affine matrix of the form

$$\Omega_{i,k}\begin{pmatrix} n_1 \\ n_2 \\ \cdot \\ n_i \\ n_k \\ 1 \end{pmatrix} \overset{\text{def}}{\equiv} \left(\begin{pmatrix} 1 & 0 & 0 & 0 & 0 & 0 \\ 0 & 1 & 0 & 0 & 0 & 0 \\ \cdot & \cdot & \cdot & \cdot & \cdot & \cdot \\ 0 & 0 & 1 & 0 & 0 & 1 \\ 0 & 0 & 0 & 0 & 1 & -1 \\ 0 & 0 & 0 & 0 & 0 & 1 \end{pmatrix} \begin{pmatrix} n_1 \\ n_2 \\ \cdot \\ n_i \\ n_k \\ 1 \end{pmatrix} \right) = \begin{pmatrix} n_1 \\ n_2 \\ \cdot \\ n_i + 1 \\ n_k - 1 \\ 1 \end{pmatrix} \tag{10}$$

on the set of coordinates of the state point. The consistent application of the shift operator of N^* times ensures a transition from one segment of length $N^*$to the next segment of the length N^* in the state space. In a symbolic space, such a transition for N^*steps will correspond to a sequence of matrices of the form.

$$\Omega_{N^*} \overset{\text{def}}{\equiv} \left(\prod_{1}^{N*} \Omega_{i,k} \right) \; for \; \forall(i, k) \tag{11}$$

The N^*-fold multiplication of the matrices Ω_{N^*} determines the matrix of frequency for each elementary transition and, accordingly, the transition probabilities matrix $\widehat{w}_{m,k}$.

Assuming that the transition probabilities obey the stationary properties, the prognosis is carried out as follows:

First, in a symbolic space, the problem of the wandering of a point for N^* elementary steps is formulated. Further constructions of model and prediction algorithms have many options, and this set is determined by the characteristics of the observed signal as sequences of indexed N and fixed triple of remaining indices. These properties include the Markov property, stationarity, and ergodicity of each cascade of wavelet coefficients.

The presence of these properties must be checked either by direct calculations based on manipulations with wavelet decompositions or by the calculation of the entropic, dimensional (information, capacitive, dimensionality, etc.) characteristics of the observed trajectories, their correlation radius. In addition, it is necessary to analyze the conditions of point-wise Hölder regularity of the observed and predicted trajectory on the basis of two microlocalizations.

Thus, the vector $(n_1, \dots n_k)$ is defined as the internal state of the automaton, and this vector corresponds to the frequency histogram of the vector $\left\{ {}^{k}_{Hist}W^{N;N=1,2,3,\dots,N^*}_{i,j} \right\} \subset R^{N^*}$, Matrix operator $\boldsymbol{\Omega}_{N^*}$ determines the transition frequencies. If to move from frequency representations to probabilistic standard renormalization $(n_i \to p_i)$, then the evolution equation for p_i looks as follows in the continuous representation in time:

$$\frac{\partial p_m}{\partial t} = \sum_k \left[\widehat{w}_{k,m} p_k - \widehat{w}_{m,k} p_m\right] \tag{12}$$

where $\widehat{w}_{k,m}$ is the transition probabilities defined by the operator $\boldsymbol{\Omega}_{N^*}$. Eq. (12) is the so-called kinetic equation, the master equation or, by its nature, the balance Equation [18]. The change in the internal state of the automaton is described by the solution of Eq. (12). On the other hand, the change in the internal state of automaton is defined as the walk of a point along $N^* - 1$ dimensional simplex Σ^{N^*-1}, defined by condition $\sum_i n_i = N^*$ and transitions $\Omega_{i,k}$ are defined on the one-dimensional faces of the simplex.

The solution of Eq. (12) gives sufficient information for solving the problem of random walk in the space $\boldsymbol{W} \stackrel{\text{def}}{=} \left\{ {}^{k}_{Hist} W^{N}_{i,j} \right\}$ in the representation of the probabilities of the transition from one vector of space to another in the form of a Feynman path integral. In many cases, to implement the tasks of the prognosis и and time estimates of reaching the boundary of the region of cardiac events, it is only sufficient to solve Eq. (12), that is, the solution of the problem of a walk on the simplex Σ^{N^*-1}. This is possible in cases where the early predictors are expressed in the singularities of walking on the simplex Σ^{N^*-1}. As in the space of trajectories, such predictors distinguish regions of the simplex for such predictors.

However, in the space formed by the cascade wavelet coefficients of the ECG, from the construction itself follows that in the normal operation of the heart in the transition from one state vector to another, the solution of equation must be stationary, if not for all cascades, then for some subset of them. Taking into account biological rhythms and other cyclic processes in the body from experimental tests, it follows that in fact the solutions of Eq. (12) satisfy the stationarity condition (13) in the "average"

$$\widehat{w}_{k,m} = \sum_m \widehat{w}_{m,k} \tag{13}$$

That is, fluctuations of the stationary solution whose amplitude is determined from the chronological database are allowed. Thus, the loss of stability of the stationary solution with subsequent transitions to another stationary solution changes the nature of a walk in space $\boldsymbol{W}$ and leads the trajectory to the boundary of the region of cardiac events. In this case, the nature of the fluctuations and their amplitude varies, and the analogy of such changes is the dynamics of the fluctuations during phase transitions. In addition, this is only one of the prognosis scenarios. Another scenario corresponds to the violation of the stationarity conditions and the time-dependent solutions of Eq. (12). This scenario will be discussed in the next section.

In conclusion, a few words about early predictors are discussed. In order for this class of predictors not to be empty, it suffices to point out violations of stationarity conditions and conditions of point-wise Holder regularity, in particular, on the change of Holder exponent of the ECG signal at the time t_0. The conditions for such events, the so-called two-microlocal conditions, are also defined on the wavelet coefficients [17] and, consequently, are present in space in the form of regions determined by various kinds of inequalities that limit the set of admissible values of wavelet coefficients.

Let us give some examples. When the stationarity condition is satisfied, the prediction problem reduces to the problem of the wandering of point on the multidimensional lattice Z^n. Here, the method of constructing a symbolic space allows to correctly move to the continuous model and uses the technique Feynman path integral. In this case, the probability of reaching a pre-assigned point of symbolic or basic state space is estimated. The time estimates in terms of the number of elementary steps to achieve a pre-determined state are given subsequently. These states also include the ranges of values of wavelet coefficients that do not satisfy the conditions of homogeneous or point-wise Hölder regularity. As can be seen from the formulas, the estimates vary depending on the characteristics of the observed ECG signal or its wavelet coefficients. For example, if the effect of excluded volume is taken into account, when forbidden trajectories appear in a set of admissible trajectories. Such a phenomenon is possible when the fragments of the cardiac myocyte sequences are turned off as a result of local myocardial degradation, when groups of conducting cardiac myocytes no longer can fully or partially perform their conductive functions. The effect of excluded volume significantly changes the properties of the considered processes.

For example, the Chapman-Kolmogorov equation becomes unjust, the system is no longer a Markovian system, and so on. Such phenomena on the one hand are themselves predictors; on the other hand, for correct estimates, it is necessary to introduce the transition probabilities and PDF containing more variables.

In this situation, the change in the properties of a myocardial tissue is associated with the discrepancy between the observed and predicted ECG parameters of the wavelet coefficients, which is a signal for automatic complication of the model by the birth of new automata. In concrete example, the appearance of forbidden trajectories (the effect of excluded volume) is a command to construct three-dimensional histograms and multidimensional transition functions. However, the further principles of the operation of automata remain unchanged. The same multiplication of automata can occur at searching for hidden predictors. For example, in estimating the change in the properties of regularity, smoothness, and so on, trajectories as a criterion are often inequalities that contain sums over the time index j.

Thus, when the stationarity conditions are fulfilled, the prognosis is reduced to estimates to reach the critical regions by a trajectory or a class of trajectories. Depending on the characteristics of the process, the estimate may vary, and a correction of the prognosis is necessary. It is this fact that determines the monitoring regimes, their frequency, and duration. In this case, the degree of deviation of the observed trajectory from the predicted trajectory, or its characteristics: moments, properties, conditions of Holder, and so on, is also estimated.

If the quasi-stationary conditions are violated at the first step, taking into account the trends of transition probabilities, a new PDF is determined on the basis of the kinetic equation; then, taking into account the changes in the PDF and the trends of transition probabilities, trajectories or their new characteristics are recalculated. However, under the conditions of fulfilling the quasi-stationary conditions, a change in the structure of the transition probabilities, an increase in the amplitude of their fluctuations, and a change in the structure of the set of transition functions are possible. In this case, the algorithms calculate the change in the positions of the values in the space of the PDF approximation parameters, their proximity to the bifurcation set. Taking into account the approach speed of the approximation parameters with the bifurcation set, a further prediction in the state space is corrected. Trajectories in this case means a set of trajectories in a set of spaces, and the earliest signs can appear for the coefficients of only one class of trajectories with a fixed triplet of indices. Subsequently, predictors can appear on the remaining classes of trajectories with other fixed indices.

5. Interaction with devices

The interaction of the remote monitoring system with implantable and portable devices is built according to the following scheme:

1. Initially, there is a set of statistical data in a chronological database. In view of the peculiarities of the set of statistics, it is necessary that the samples for all fixed indices be representative both at rest and in the state of motion.
2. At such set, the automata create a database of valid trajectories in small dimensions.
3. With the full set of chronological database, automata begin calculations according to the algorithms described earlier.

The further mode of preventive monitoring is determined by automata and is based on the requirement of sufficiency of statistics. After that, the automata determine the further monitoring strategy. During the operation of automata, numerous additional hidden predictors are identified, the earliest. If the development of hidden predictors leads to the emergence and development of existing predictors, a minimal subclass is allocated as signal and management automata from the whole class of automata. Their volume should correspond to small computing resources of implantable or portable devices. Further, this minimal subset is transferred to the device's memory and further serves as a signal device that controls the calculations on the remote server. The described scenario allows to optimize costs and the preventive monitoring modes.

6. Verification

The experimental verification of the capabilities of the set of recognizing automata presented in this chapter is carried out continuously during the last 4 years [19–21]. The ECG signal is selected as an initial observed signal for the analysis and prediction of cardiac events. The standard scheme for measuring the ECG signal by a recorder in 12 leads with a variable sampling rate of 1–2 kHz and a 24-bit resolution is considered.

The wearable ECG set has DSP compute block on-board to partially offload cloud infrastructure and to monitor cardio events in real time. The particular set of automata computed locally depends on power demand-reaction time tradeoff, which in turn depends on particular patient's case. In any case, all the collected data are compressed and transferred to the cloud.

Currently, Wi-Fi is used for communication. Mobile connectivity in spaces where Wi-Fi infrastructure is not present is achieved via mobile Wi-Fi tethering with smartphone (mostly to get rid of multiple sim cards burden). Also, the device carries Bluetooth LE which is used for settings transfer and standard on-site real-time monitoring via tablet software or PC software if one carries BLE receiver. A schematic diagram of the cluster work is presented in **Figure 4**.

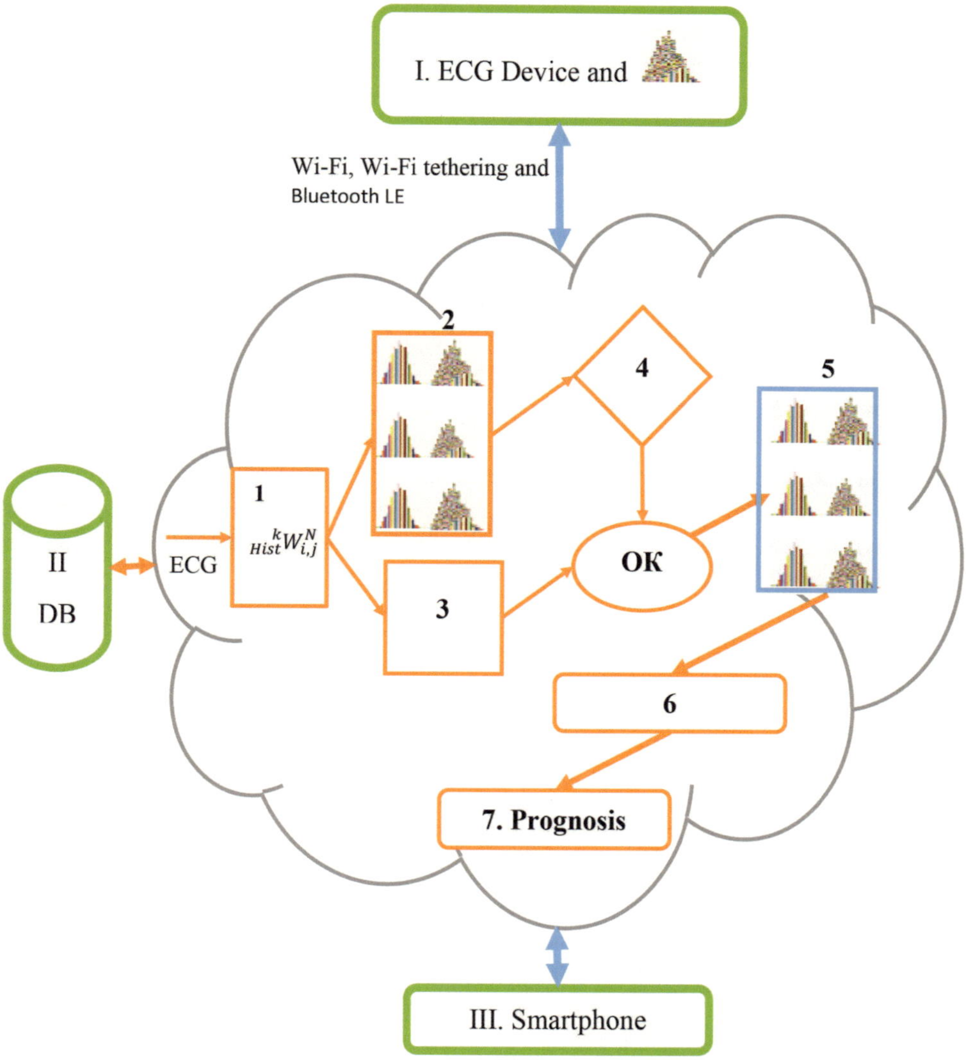

Figure 4. A schematic diagram of work of remote preventive cardiac-monitoring cluster: ECG device and on-board recognizing automata for the realization of signal function and management by recognizing automata in the cloud (I); database, chronological database of patient, database of HE (II); smartphone for text-graphic messages of cluster (III); 1—space W; 2—the set of interacting automata parallel to the processing of W-cascades and defining $\widehat{w}_{k,m}$; 3—two-microlocal analysis; 4—check of the quasi-stationarity; 5—prognosis in the symbolic space Σ^{N^*-1} using automata from block 2; 6—check of stability of the prognosis; 7—constructing the prognosis in the state space W.

The check consists of two stages. At the first stage, a chronological ECG database for patients is used to predict cardiac events. In doing so, the ECG is used both for cardiac events and for the ECG of the control group. Chronological databases of patients with a long history from the occurrence of cardiac events, and their subsequent treatment of drug or catheter ablation were also used. Monitoring was carried out both before ablation and after it during a long period of drug support. At the first stage of checking, the effectiveness of recognizing automata and the ability of automata to predict cardiac events were tested. In those cases when the automata did not predict a cardiac event, the automata returned to the beginning of the recording, they became more complicated, and the process was repeated. It should be noted that the main purpose of the described experiments and the basic principles laid down in the algorithms of automata are aimed at preventive monitoring, that is, on the detection of the earliest predictors of cardiac events with subsequent time estimate of the evolution of these predictors until the appearance of later predictors, already known, such as dispersion QT interval, P wave index, increased QT interval duration, and so on. The main problem, because of which there were gaps of cardiac events by automata, is as follows. If to analyze the results of each automaton individually, then during the evolution of their states, there was no approximation of the state trajectory to the boundaries of the regions of cardiac events in any of the selected metrics, but the event was happening. The analysis showed that the predictor of the event in these situations is not a violation of the quasi-stationary conditions, but a change or a mismatch in the structure of transition probabilities for some subset of automata. The revealed mismatch can be characterized in terms of conditional entropy. Ultimately, conditionally entropic characteristics were used in the approximation of conditional K-complexity, since the calculation of K-complexity is an algorithmically unsolvable problem. Another way to solve the problem is to reduce the complexity of automata in dimension, which has an analogy in the transition from single-particle PDF to multiparticle PDF.

Figure 5 shows changes in the states of automata under the action of the operator $\Omega_{N^*} = \left(\prod_{1}^{N*} \Omega_{i,k}\right)$ considered in Section 3. The figure reflects the mixing nature of the actions of the operator Ω_{N^*} and the temporal evolution of transition functions, entropic, informational, and dimensional characteristics of which determine the earliest predictors.

By changing the consistency of the state trajectories of a certain subset of automata, it is implied in this case that early predictors are defined as differences in the structure of operators

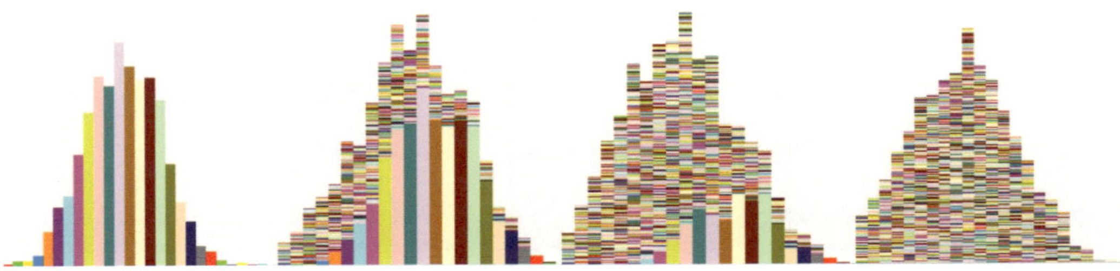

Figure 5. Changes in the states of automata.

Ω_{N^*}. However, here we are talking about the earliest predictors or automata, distinguishing trajectories, leading to cardiac events from trajectories without cardiac events.

If to consider traditional predictors associated with the estimation of the duration of intervals, the characteristics of the QRS complex of the alteration, P- wave, dispersion of P-wave index, then in this case, the automata predict rather successfully the evolution of the listed predictors.

This is important for drug treatment of persistent AF and optimization of drug therapy, as for many other cardiac applications.

7. Task of management of the trajectories

We now return to discuss the management problem mentioned in Section "Introduction." The set of admissible trajectories is sufficiently variable. Depending on many factors, these changes are associated with cardiovascular degradation, changes in conductivity at cell scales, changes in the architecture of a set of conductive paths between sets of conducting cells, and so on. The very set of trajectories is so factorized into equivalence classes, regarding the action of groups of process symmetries, the type of the PDF process, and the set of transition probabilities. In view of the factors mentioned earlier, there are prohibitions on transitions from one state P to another. Thus, some trajectories in classes become forbidden when all these factors are taken into account, or the probability of some trajectories becomes small.

In fact, the task of controlling trajectories reduces to changing the class of trajectory or to the task of keeping a trajectory in a given class by means of variable management parameters. The management parameters include all parameters on the macro- and microlevel, which can be varied in various ways. Such methods include drug therapy with AF-AT events, and AV and VV programming of the CRT device [22, 23]. The same goals are pursued with ablation or defibrillation. Within the framework of the presented model, all possible ways to change the class of trajectories to the class of trajectories that do not terminate HE are formalized as shown in **Figure 6**, where the management loop is mapped into a state space or trajectories.

Passing to formal language of homotopy theory and theory of infinite loop spaces [24], the process of management defined by the mapping

$$S : \partial I^{k+1} \to \partial C^k \tag{14}$$

k + 1 is the dimension cube, k is the number of management parameters, k + 1 is the parameter —time.

At each fixed time t and with the variations of other κ parameters, a mapping the boundary of k—dimension cube to the area homotopically equivalent k-dimensional sphere in K is defined

$$S^- : \partial I^k \to \partial C^k \subset K \tag{15}$$

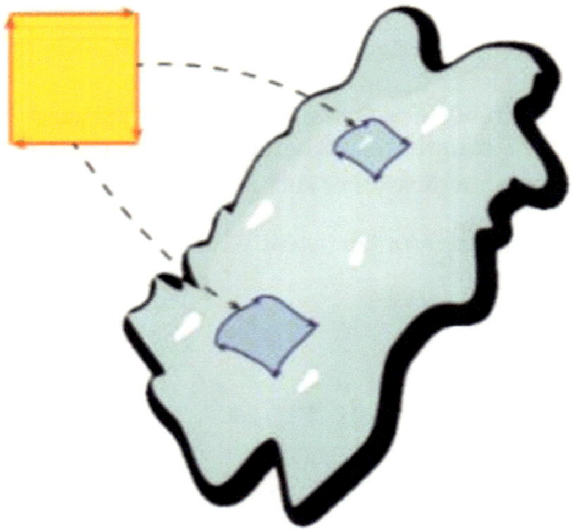

Figure 6. Management loop (yellow color) is mapped into a state space of trajectories (blue color).

Definition 1.

The management task is solvable if and only if.

1. The set of homotopy classes $\left[\partial I^k,\ \partial C^k\right]$ is trivial or.

2. The mapping S^- belongs to the trivial element of the set of homotopy classes.

In these examples, the set of homotopy classes has a group structure and is defined as the k-homotopy group of the k-dimensional sphere $\left[\partial I^k, \partial C^k\right] = \pi_k\left(\partial C^k\right)$.

In other words, the management problem is solvable if, with the help of a variation of management parameters, the observed trajectory can be deformed into a predefined trajectory if and only if there is no forbidden trajectory or other topological obstacles between them. A little more optimism is given by the following statement: if the management problem is not solvable with this set of management parameters, then changing the number of management-led parameters can possibly translate the problem into a class of solvable management problems. In the version of recognizing automata, the management problem and the calculation of the management strategy are reduced to determining the influence of the management parameters on the set of admissible transition probabilities in the predefined class of trajectories.

8. Conclusion

Several years of experimenting with recognizing automata and the preliminary obtained results allow to make optimistic conclusions about preventive medicine, in particular, preventive monitoring. The development of mHealth platforms, portable and implantable devices, on-body sensors, and so on, available wireless data transmission systems and available computing power allow solving very complex prognosis in a very short time and in a number of cases in real time. Thus, the development of preventive monitoring systems creates a trend toward changing paradigms, at least in the field of cardiology. If early predictors exist, then a natural question arises, but is there any possibility of influencing the character and speed of development of early, preventive predictors via preventive drug therapy, different diets, and so on in the direction of reversibility of the current situation. That is, does the class of trajectories exist when early appeared predictors are eliminated by preventive maintenance, otherwise when the situation is physically reversible? In the PHM/IMS applications to technical objects, the term "self-maintenance, self-recovery" appears. Medicine is more conservative, and yet the above analogy is appropriate. In the context of preventive cardiomonitoring, this means that the number of age groups that preventive control is recommended increases markedly and begins on average from 30 to 40 years. This is also indicated by the statistics of the growth of heart diseases, which currently has the nature of a pandemic, as well as statistics on the rejuvenation of heart diseases [25]. The concrete ways of creating preventive monitoring systems are now quite realistic and are reduced to the realization of the fact that the chronological basis of the individual's ECG data is needed to identify early predictors.

The database is updated periodically. The question of the refresh rate is solved by the system of recognizing automata.

Author details

Sergey Kirillov[1]*, Aleksandr Kirillov[1], Vitalii Iakimkin[1], Michael Pecht[2] and Yuri Kaganovich[3]

*Address all correspondence to: skirillovru@gmail.com

1 SmartSys Prognosis Center, Moscow, Russia

2 Center for Advanced Life Cycle Engineering, University of Maryland, Maryland, USA

3 Department of Cardiology, Assuta Medical Center, Tel Aviv, Israel

References

[1] Martirosyan M, Caliskan K, Theuns D, Szili-Torok T. Remote monitoring of heart failure: Benefits for therapeutic decision making. Expert Review of Cardiovascular Therapy. 2017; **15**(7). DOI: DOI.org/10.1080/14779072.2017.1348229

[2] Lerma C, Glass L. Predicting the risk of sudden cardiac death. The Journal of Physiology. 2016;**594**(9):2445-2458. DOI: 10.1113/JP270535

[3] Piotrowicz E. The management of patients with chronic heart failure: The growing role of e-health, journal. Expert Review of Medical Devices. 2017;**14**(4). DOI: 10.1080/17434440.2017.1314181

[4] Luther S, Fenton F, Kornreich B, et al. low-energy control of electrical turbulence in the heart. Nature. 2011;**475**(7355):235-239. DOI: 10.1038/nature10216

[5] Lin J, Keener J. Microdomain effects on transverse cardiac propagation. Biophysical Journal. 2014;**106**(4):925-931

[6] Bressloff P. Stochastic Processes in Cell Biology. Cham: Springer; 2014. DOI: 10.1007/978-3-319-08488-6

[7] Ugarte JP, Orozco-Duque A, Tobón C, et al. Dynamic approximate entropy electroanatomic maps detect rotors in a simulated atrial fibrillation model. PLoS ONE. 2014. DOI: 10.1371/journal.pone.0114577

[8] Kleinert H. Path Integrals in Quantum Mechanics, Statistics, Polymer Physics, and Financial Markets. Singapore/River Edge: World ScientificVenecia; 2004

[9] Ziman J. Model of Disorder. Cambridge: Cambridge University Press; 1979

[10] Boles U, Enriquez A, Abdollah H, Michael K. Early changes on the electrocardiogram in hypertension. E-Journal of the ESC Council for Cardiology Practice. 08 Sep 2015;**13**(N°30)

[11] Martinez A, Alcaraz R, Rieta JJ. Study on the P-wave feature time course as early predictors of paroxysmal atrial fibrillation. Physiological Measurement. 2012;**33**(12):1959-1974

[12] Kleber A, Rudy Y. Basic mechanisms of cardiac impulse propagation and associated arrhythmias. Physiological Reviews. 2004;**84**:431-488. DOI: 10.1152/physrev.00025.2003

[13] Potse M, Dube B, Richer J, Vinet A, Gulrajani R. A comparison of monodomain and bidomain reaction-diffusion models for action potential propagation in the human heart. IEEE Transactions on Biomedical Engineering. 2006;**53**(12):2425-2435

[14] Keizer J. Statistical Thermodynamics of Nonequilibrium Processes. Berlin: Springer; 1987

[15] Husemoller D. Fibre Bundles. New York: Springer. DOI: 10.1007/978-1-4757-2261-1

[16] Horsthemke W, Lefever R. Theory and Applications in Physics, Chemistry,and Biology. Berlin Heibelberg New York: Springer; 1984

[17] Jaffard S, Meyer Y. Wavelet methods for pointwise regularity and local oscillations of functions. Memorirs of American Mathematical Society. 1996;**123**:N587

[18] Nicolis G, Prigogine I. Self-Organization in Nonequilibrium Systems: From Dissipative Structures to Order through Fluctuations. New York: A Wiley-Interscience Publication; 1977

[19] Kirillov S, Kirillov A, Iakimkin V, Khodos F, Kaganovich Y, Pecht M. PHM applications in medicine and medical implantable device. In: Prognostics and System Health Management Conference (PHM-Chengdu); 2016. DOI: 10.1109/PHM.2016.7819755

[20] Kaganovich Y, Kirillov S. Remote PHM cloud cluster for Arrhtyhmia prognosis and drug control efficient. Journal of Atrial Fibrillation. 2013, Speical Issue

[21] Kaganovich Y, Kirillov S, Kirillov A. Remote PHM cloud cluster for heart failure prognosis and drug therapy optimization: First results. EP – Europace. 2015;**17**(S2):132

[22] Bradham W, Gold M. The role of AV and VV optimization for CRT. Journal of Arrhythmia. 2013;**29**(3):153-161. DOI: 10.1016/j.joa.2013.02.001

[23] Nawar A, El-Hoseiny R, Ragab D, Al-Aziz A. V–V delay interval optimization in CRT using echocardiography compared to QRS width in surface ECG. The Egyptian Heart Journal. September 2012;**64**(3):127-133. DOI: 10.1016/j.ehj.2011.08.013

[24] Adams J. Infinite Loop Spaces. Princeton: Princeton Universiry Press; 1978

[25] Anter E, Jessup M, Callans D. Atrial fibrillation and heart failure treatment considerations for a dual epidemic. Circulation. 2009;**119**:2516-2525. DOI: /10.1161/CIRCULATIONAHA.108.821306